Read My Plate

Read My Plate

The Literature of Food

Deborah R. Geis

LEXINGTON BOOKS
Lanham • Boulder • New York • London

Published by Lexington Books
An imprint of The Rowman & Littlefield Publishing Group, Inc.
4501 Forbes Boulevard, Suite 200, Lanham, Maryland 20706
www.rowman.com

6 Tinworth Street, London SE11 5AL

British Library Cataloguing in Publication Information Available

Library of Congress Cataloging-in-Publication Data Available

ISBN 978-1-4985-7443-3 (cloth : alk. paper)
ISBN 978-1-4985-7445-7 (pbk: alk. paper)
ISBN 978-1-4985-7444-0 (electronic)

∞™ The paper used in this publication meets the minimum requirements of American National Standard for Information Sciences Permanence of Paper for Printed Library Materials, ANSI/NISO Z39.48-1992.

Contents

Acknowledgments

Chapter 4 ("Feeding the Audience: Food, Feminism, and Performance Art") appeared in an earlier form in *Eating Culture*, edited by Ron Scapp and Brian Seitz (Albany: SUNY Press, 1998). Grateful acknowledgment is made to the editors and press for permission to adapt.

Photographs (cover and figure 1) are by Hamish Gavin; used with permission.

Thanks to Lindsey Falk, Jessica Thwaite, and the editorial team at Lexington Books for believing in this project and providing superb guidance.

So many of my present and former colleagues at DePauw University have made a tremendous difference in my work on this book. I want particularly to thank English Department secretary extraordinaire Annie Weltz for her constant support, and my colleagues Samuel Autman, Mike Sinowitz, and Wayne Glausser for their unflagging food enthusiasm. I also thank Meryl Altman, David Alvarez, Beth Benedix, Harry Brown, John Caraher, Tom Chiarella, Istvan Csicsery-Ronay, Vanessa Dickerson, Emily Doak, Dana Dudle, Ron Dye, Gigi Jennewein Fenlon, Angela Flury, Eugene Gloria, Caroline Good, Tim Good, Peter Graham, Susan Hahn, Kelley Hall, Amy Hayes, Andrew Hayes, Tiffany Hebb, Joe Heithaus, Lynn Ishikawa, Jeannette Johnson-Licon, Hillary Kelleher, Bobbi Kelley, Kevin Kinney, Marnie McInnes, Claudia Mills, Jonathan Nichols-Pethick, Keith Nightenhelser, Veronica Pejril, Amity Reading, Pamela Kay Roberts, Greg Schwipps, Karen Singson, Mike Sinowitz, Alicia Suarez, Andrea Sununu, Tamara Stasik, Chris White, Karin Wimbley, David Worthington, and Lili Wright.

My oldest friends—from high school, college, grad school, and Knoxville and New York City years—mean everything to me, and I thank them here: Maura Ann Abrahamson, Jonathan Allison, Beth Baldwin, Anna Battigelli, Anthony Barone, Barbara Bowen, Glenn Burger, Ava Chin, Tracy and Reinold Cornelius, Jay Dickson, John Evelev, Lynda Finn, Billy Finnegan, Mary and Stephan Flores, Jonathan and Lara Frater, Angelique Garner, Debbie Grove, George Held, Emily Jones, Marilyn Kallet, Cynthia Koch, Steven F. Kruger, Ed Ku, Leslie LaChance, Joyce Ann McGinn, James Magruder, Lisa Suhair Majaj, David Mikics, Wayne Moreland, Kathleen Moore, Diana Marcus Muller, Tony O'Brien, Julie Olin-Ammentorp, Warren Olin-Ammentorp, Franny Osman, Lee Papa, Janet Pennisi, Claudia Petersen, Adam Potkay, Lloyd Andrew Roberts,

Evan Ross, Ilana Saraf, Ron Scapp, Peter Schamel, Len Schiff, Chari Smith, Emily Smith, Don Summa, Elizabeth Sutherland, James Tulsky, Robert Vorlicky, Karen J. Vrotsos, Ann Frank Wake, Chuck Wasserburg, John Weir, David J. Weiss, and Regina Rousso Wilmes.

This book also would never have happened without the daily sustenance and humor that I have found in my online community. Some of them are also inspired and inspiring cooks: Jennifer Burns Bright, Eliza Kaufman Gross, Ariel Lopez, Mitchell Lord, Chris McManus, Lucinda Gwendolyn Rothchild (in her own way), Stephen Shapiro, Erin Elizabeth Smith, Jack Verde, and Eric Wiener. There are too many who make me smile every single day to mention them all, but I especially thank Fred Aaron, Rich Appel, Alicia Bailey, Rob Broder, Aimee Cegelka, Matthew Cordell, Jeff Damal, Cris Diaz, Marvin B. Edmiston, Sheila Ellis, Shawn Marie Garrett, Jeffrey Gillis, David Hale, Erin Hemmer, Mica Hilson, Fritz Liess, Holland MacFallister, Ron Malott, David Mendez, David Hamilton Neely, Gene O'Brien, David Roberson, Paul Senules, Edward Shaw, Dean Squibb, Matt Sumpter, Michael Angelo Tata, Michael Venable, and Baju Wijono.

Special thanks to my sisters, their husbands, and my three nephews for sharing more meals with me than I can possibly count, and for their ongoing love and support: Nancy Geis Bardgett, Sarah Geis Williams, Mark Bardgett, Timothy Scott Williams, Caleb D. Bardgett, Will Badgett, and Benjamin Jordan Bardgett. My mother, Dorothy Geis, passed away before I completed this book. She and my late friend Carlos A. Marsh, who also loved food, were always in my thoughts as I worked on this volume.

My greatest thanks are reserved for Hamish Gavin and for the joy that he has brought to my life. A conversation about pizza turned into this book and so much more. This book is dedicated to him (and to Cara, Cocoa, and Trigger for helping me write it).

Introduction

In recent years, an astounding array of writing about food has been published. From reissues of M.F.K. Fisher's classic memoir/cookbook hybrids (collected in *The Art of Eating*) to Ruth Reichl's autobiographical trilogy that began with *Tender at the Bone*, to Diana Abu-Jaber's *The Language of Baklava*, among many others, powerful works of creative nonfiction in which an author presents his or her past through a focus on eating and cooking have made their way into the literary marketplace. At the same time in the academic arena, perhaps due in part to the popularity of so-called OOOT (Object-Oriented Ontological Theory, which gives primacy to the "things" in culture), critics are starting to reread works of fiction, drama, and poetry by paying close attention to how and what the characters cook and eat. In *Read My Plate: The Literature of Food*, I look at food writing in both fictional and nonfictional genres. My thesis is that not only does an attention to food often subvert traditional narrative expectations (in, for example, the inclusion of recipes, which we "read" differently from other prose), but it also provides crucial forms of access to memory and emotion that might otherwise be repressed. From the politics of gluttony to the politics of aging, food is always part of an intensified set of experiences that can serve (as in the case of school lunches) as forms of alienation/confrontation through religion, race, culture, or gender.

The discipline of literary "food studies" has become increasingly popular in academia through the work of scholars like Sandra Gilbert, Megan Elias, Henry Notaker, Priscilla Parkhurst Ferguson, and many others, and in a larger context through the work of food journalists like Eric Schlosser and Michael Pollan. However, while many of us teach courses about the literature of food, food as it appears within literary texts (fiction, poetry, the graphic novel, drama) and as it appears in creative nonfiction (the food memoir) has not been treated as a unified subject of textual study, and to do so is my intention in this volume. The goals of this book are threefold: (a) to explore ways that narrative form and readerly response are affected by giving eating/cooking a primary place in a work; (b) to amplify connections between the cultural identities of characters or narrators and their "food lives"; and (c) to provide evidence that both acts—reading literary works "through" food, and reading memoirs "about" food from a literary standpoint—richly expand our traditional approaches to textual interpretation. My premise, then, is that the kind of close reading available through examining how and what narrators or

characters cook and eat—in effect, through reading their "plates"—
creates a powerful, visceral means of textual analysis.

I imagine the rest of this introductory chapter to be like the cook's
mise-en-place, the station where he or she sets out the ingredients to be
used in the preparation of a dish. In this case, my *mise-en-place* has six
components. In order to illustrate my personal connection to this project,
I begin with an example of how I might go about "reading" my own plate
of food. From there, I consider why, beyond the obvious idea that we
need it to live, we are so fascinated by food, and how its scrutiny helps us
to understand contemporary culture, literature, and identity politics. I
then begin the turn from food itself to food writing, with an emphasis on
why we should pay attention to it, and why M.F.K. Fisher was such an
important influence on how such writing is done. The following section
explores ways that food writing treats issues of narrative voice, particularly with the inclusion of recipes. I discuss how the recent critical interest in the philosophy of "things" (OOOT) amplifies the way we think
about food. And the final ingredient of my introduction is a brief over-
view of the upcoming chapters.

WHAT'S ON MY PLATE?: CONSIDER THE TOURTIÈRE

Before I became involved with a Canadian man, I never really knew that
Canadians eat differently than the way Americans do. When they order
French fries, they ask for gravy on the side, even when they are not eating
poutine. They eat poutine, and something called smoked meat. Their
airport souvenir stands have little bottles of maple syrup with a Canadian flag on the label. And perhaps by some kind of law, they have to
stop at a place called Tim Horton's and drink a beverage called a "dou-
ble-double" or an "ice cap" every two hours. I already knew about the
poutine and the smoked meat, and I had been to Tim Horton's in Ontario
a couple of times back in the day, but what surprised me most was that
although I thought I knew my exotic foodstuffs pretty well, I had never
heard of tourtière—before last August, which is apparently not the time
that one normally eats tourtière, but the Canadian man and I had gotten
in the habit of asking one another what we were having for dinner, and
he said that he had just put a frozen tourtière in the oven. As with some
of his British-inflected expressions that I didn't understand but was too
embarrassed to ask, I had to Google it. I knew that "tortue" meant "tor-
toise" in French, but surely he wasn't eating turtle. And so I learned
something, and I knew I had to try it.

The first things I learned about tourtière were from Wikipedia: it orig-
inates from Québécois culture, is a popular dish for Canadians to have
after midnight mass on Christmas Eve or on New Year's Eve, and you
can find it year-round in the frozen food department of grocery stores

throughout Canada. There's so much more to it than that, though, even including controversies over the origins of its name and how best to prepare it. The website allrecipes.com defines tourtière as a "double-crusted meat pie with a savory pork, beef, onion and spice filling. A delicious, fragrant and savory addition to the holiday table." The spices that give it its unique (and Christmassy) flavor might typically include cinnamon, clove, allspice, and nutmeg. Different regions of Canada offer other types of tourtière with varying fillings, though, including some that feature wild game or even salmon. In Saguenay-Lac-Saint-Jean and eastern Québec, the filling has cubed potatoes in it; in Montréal, they make it with pork and eat it with a sweet condiment like maple syrup, cranberry compote, or tomato chutney; in St. Boniface and rural French-speaking parts of Manitoba, they have their signature spice mixture; in New Brunswick, Novia Scotia, and Prince Edward Island, they use pork but may also include chicken, rabbit, or beef.

According to food historian Nathalie Cooke in *What's to Eat? Entrées in Canadian Food History*, the precursor of the tourtière seems to have been the "sea pie" (a pun or heard-invention from the French "cipaille") which was a portable meat pie that eighteenth century sailors carried with them in a cauldron in order not to have to eat only fish on their voyages (Cooke 2009, 109). Many culinary writers who are interested in the history of pie—and who wouldn't be?—have pointed out that meat pies go back at least as far as 1600 BCE Mesopotamia (see Peyton 2018 et al.). Sasha Chapman writes that the word "tourte" probably comes from the Latin slang term *tortus panis*, meaning a round of bread, though some would claim (perhaps erroneously) that it is related not to turtles, but to pigeons, as the French word for "pigeon" is also "tourte," and pigeons were probably sometimes caught and baked into these pies, though this probably isn't where their name comes from. The tourtière, then, is most likely named for the deep-dish vessel in which one bakes this "tourte." Chapman adds that what may be the first French-Canadian cookbook, *La Cuisinière Canadienne*, published several recipes for tourtière in 1840, and she quotes another food historian, Elizabeth Driver, who points out that although tourtières are now made with ground meat, the original versions of them would have used meat that was cut into small pieces with a knife (Chapman 2018).

Food blogger Rachel Arsenault, who grew up among many French-Canadian immigrants in a small New England town, writes, "Almost every family had a tante or memère (aunt or grandmother) who had a tourtière recipe with a secret ingredient or two" (Arsenault 2015). Gabby Peyton remarks in her entry on tourtière for Food Bloggers of Canada, "It's not a dish for one; it's always eaten with friends and family" (Peyton 2018). Amongst these friends and family members, apparently, whose tourtière is the best can become quite a competitive sport. Lynn Neary of National Public Radio, in her piece on the dish for "The Salt," recalls having been at Canadian Christmastime events where rival cooks in a family vied for the recognition of having made the superior tourtière, and she quotes Thomas Naylor, who at the time was executive chef to the Canadian ambassador to the United States, as saying, "it's like hockey rivalry" (Neary 2011). (Ah, yes, hockey. Another whole subject I learned about.)

That's what I was able to find out, but of course, I still wanted to know more—and to taste it myself. I finally had the chance to do so in January 2018, upon a much-anticipated visit to Winnipeg to see the Canadian man. But I didn't get to try some grandmother's version of the dish—rather, perhaps more appropriately for this project, I first tried tourtière at a bookstore—a bookstore/café, that is, called McNally Robinson. As if in celebration of the hybrid cultural identities that make up Canadian cuisine, we began the meal with a Senegalese peanut soup. And completely against the grain of the tourtière as a family dish meant to be shared, this one arrived on my plate as one small, perfect pie, designed to be eaten by an individual diner. The crust was thicker than the crust for a fruit pie; the meat filling had an almost Jamaican taste (thanks to the allspice); there was a little dish of brown gravy (instead of the sweet condiments that some serve) on the side, which I spooned onto the tourtière a little bit at a time as I ate it. Although I had been anticipating the moment of my first taste of tourtière for months, it was so rich that I couldn't finish it, and had to hand the rest of my plate over to the Canadian man.

Months later, I tried a full-size, more traditional tourtière from a place in Winnipeg called Miller's Meats, where you bring one home and bake it yourself in the oven for about an hour (no microwaving). This one had a lighter crust, though I think it was made with lard in the traditional style, and the filling had a richer mouth-feel but wasn't heavily spiced. Rather guiltily, I put some ketchup on the side (tourtière seems to require some kind of condiment to keep it moist), but wished that I had bought some chutney. And that night, I began dreaming of how I, a non-Canadian, would (once the weather got cold again) try making the perfect tourtière myself: add some ground lamb and some caramelized onions to the meat mixture; perhaps create a puff pastry crust. It wouldn't necessarily be authentic, but I would serve it with love and join in on the story.

FOOD, TRANSFORMATION, AND CULTURAL IDENTITY

Food offers, both literally (in the sense that we consume and digest it, and what and how much we eat or don't eat changes our bodies) and figuratively (in the sense that we use it for reward, for punishment [e.g., the "slop" on the CBS reality show *Big Brother*], for seduction, as a social class marker, etc.) the possibility for transformation. Food historian Felipe

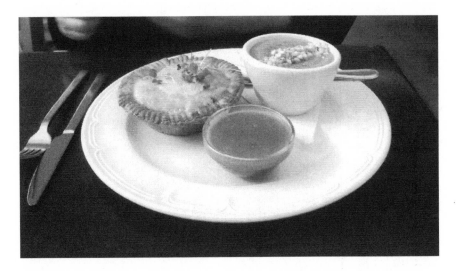

Figure 0.1. Tourtière at McNally-Robinson, Winnipeg, Canada. Photo by Hamish Gavin.

Fernández-Armesto—despite the fact that he is really talking about eating practices in the context of cannibalism!—offers a useful catalogue of some of the ways that eating is a "culturally transforming" act:

> It has its own alchemy. It transmutes individuals into society and sickness into health. It changes personalities. It can sacralize apparently secular acts. It functions like ritual. It becomes ritual. It can make food divine or diabolic. It can release power. It can create bonds. It can signify revenge or love. It can proclaim identity. A change as revolutionary as any in the history of our species happened when eating stopped being merely practical and became ritual, too. From cannibals to homeopathists and health foodies, eaters target foods which they think will burnish their characters, extend their powers, prolong their lives. (Fernández-Arnesto 2015, 345)

The way we talk and think about food, then, is really about much more than the food itself. Diana Fuss remarks, "Narratives of 'eating culture' act out complex cultural fantasies of desire and inhibition, loss and plenitude, demand and refusal, wish and fulfillment" (Fuss 1998, 237). Food is about both pleasure and danger, as Priscilla Parkhurst Ferguson reminds us: "Sometimes we about food simply to talk about food. Yet as often as not we talk *through* food to speak of love and desire, devotion and disgust, aspirations and anxieties, ideas and ideologies, joys and judgments" (Ferguson 2014, xiv). Her use of alliteration calls attention to the linked acts of eating and talking: we are conscious of orality in a new way when we pay attention to the words we choose to characterize food and our relationship to it.

We might indeed use food to claim an identity—to declare oneself a "vegan" is to take on an entire set of cultural markers, even if not all of them apply—or to acquire a certain level of social cachet (when we post on Instagram our pictures from a fancy restaurant) in the effort to be identified as "sophisticated" or as a "foodie." This identity might be strongly linked to our ethnic, religious, racial, or familial heritage as Italian, Jewish, African American, etc., as countless food memoirs and cookbooks have shown. Ferguson suggests that "[e]very act of consumption says something about the universe that we make for ourselves. A whole range of food choices engages fundamental beliefs that connect the individual to a group, a community and a country" (Ferguson 2014, 42).

At the same time, there is a kind of cultural tourism involved on an everyday basis as we decide whether to "go" Thai, Indian, or Mexican for the next meal. For the most part, what we prepare or consume may not be particularly authentic interpretations of each culture's cuisine, and writers like bell hooks and others have pointed out that eating at the local Chinese buffet doesn't give you any right to claim an investment in or knowledge of multiculturalism. As hooks says in her essay "Eating the Other: Desire and Resistance," "Within commodity culture, ethnicity becomes spice, seasoning that can liven up the dull dish that is mainstream white culture . . . The overriding fear is that cultural, ethnic, and racial differences will be continually commodified and offered up as new dishes to enhance the white palate—that the Other will be eaten, consumed, and forgotten" (hooks 1998, 181, 200). What it does imply, though, is that in postmodern culture, there's a fluid and constantly evolving set of relationships between our culinary "travel" (which, at its worst, partakes of tokenism or essentialism) and the constant desire to experience food, paradoxically, as both a source of nostalgia (connection to and longing for the past) and a way of trying more and more and more new things.

Just as food is a potential source of transformation, so, too, is the act of reading literature: we read not simply out of the desire to obtain knowledge (as we eat for the means of survival), but also out of a desire for escape, for a wider range of experiences, for empowerment, for surprise, for nostalgia, even (at times) for sexual satisfaction. And when we read about food—cooking it, eating it, sometimes not having it or encountering it problematically—we forge a connection, whether it is in the form of a literary work, a cookbook, or a memoir, between the cerebral and the visceral. Terry Eagleton points out that the notion of food as joining the literal and the metaphorical goes back at least as far as the idea of the Eucharist. He adds, "Like the poststructuralist text, food is endlessly interpretable, as gift, threat, poison, recompense barter, seduction, solidarity, suffocation" (Eagleton 2015, 446).

As Betty Fussell puts it, "Food is always image and icon as well as substance" (Fussell 2015, 441). The problem, of course, is that language inevitably falls short of the ability to convey how something tastes. Every season on the competitive show *The Next Food Network Star*, contestants (who are aspiring to host their own cooking show on the network) are castigated for using blanket words like "delicious" instead of coming up with more powerfully descriptive adjectives to convey to the audience what a dish tastes like. Ferguson reminds us that visual images in magazines and on video attempt to bring us closer to the actual experience of eating (Ferguson 2014, 44), which is also an aphorism we hear incessantly on the Food Network: "you eat first with your eyes." We need, however, to be able to talk about food in order to participate in eating as a communal experience, and to do so in a way that allows us to connect food with the act of memory. Ferguson's words about the significance of the transition from talk to text when thinking about food are useful here:

> [T]o transform the individual act of eating into the social phenomenon of consumption, food talk needs texts . . . Food talk completes the culinary circuit, turning the private into the public, embellishing the personal, and memorializing the idiosyncratic . . . Like food, talk disappears . . . Texts allow . . . the comparisons that make judgment, criticism, and analysis possible . . . To have an effect beyond the individual cook or diner, cooking has to get out of the kitchen; feasting must exit the dining room. That job of conveyance to the larger food world is what food writing does. (Ferguson 2014, 50–52)

We "consume" or even "devour" a really good book; we "drink in" its contents; we read works that give us "food for thought"; we enjoy a "literary banquet." The act of reading is never too far from the act of eating—you might even be snacking on something as you are reading this. Language and food, Fussell argues, both involve using the mouth, from infancy on, to form our earliest understanding of how to negotiate between what is inside and outside of ourselves: "Even a mouth eating in solitude—and silence—is engaged willy-nilly in discovering and communing with what is outside itself, which its hunger transforms by taking the outside literally in" (Fussell 2015, 441). Or as Vertamae Smart-Grosvenor puts it in her book on soul food, *Vibration Cooking* (which will be discussed further later in this volume), "Food changes into blood, blood into cells, cells change into energy which changes up into life and since your life style is imaginative, creative, loving, energetic, serious, food is life. You dig" (Smart-Grosvenor 1992, 296).

THE CONSUMMATE FOOD WRITER: M.F.K. FISHER

Molly O'Neill notes that the term "food writer" first appeared in the *New York Times* on March 12, 1950 (O'Neill 2015, 453), and it's a term now ubiquitous in contemporary usage to cover a range of genres from restaurant reviewing to autobiographical cookbooks to food blogs and memoirs. But that date doesn't really tell the whole story. In a literary sense, we could say that "food writing" goes all the way back to Biblical times (e.g., Leviticus in the Old Testament) and to classical writers like Horace, Plutarch, and others, as Sandra Gilbert and Roger Porter have noted (Gilbert and Porter 2015, xxvi). There are more famous pivotal moments of eating in literature (the forbidden fruit in Milton's *Paradise Lost*; the cannibalistic ending of Shakespeare's *Titus Andronicus*; Proust's madeleine; the banquet in her new house that Edna Pontellier has in Kate Chopin's *The Awakening*; the *boeuf en daube* that Mrs. Ramsay serves in Virginia Woolf's *To The Lighthouse*; the plums notoriously pilfered from the icebox in William Carlos Williams's poem, to name only a few examples) than we could possibly enumerate here—and these moments have been the subject of close readings.

Despite the proliferation of these literary food scenes, it was not always acceptable to talk and write about what one was eating. As Gilbert discusses in *The Culinary Imagination*, writers like M.F.K. Fisher were "transgressive" in transforming what members of so-called polite society would want to read, given that the kitchen was a place for the lower class and that "it wasn't even proper to discuss the menu at the early twentieth-century American table" (Gilbert 2014, 146). Gilbert links the growing popularity of the food memoir as genre not only to the rise of novels that included a "frequent focus on the quotidian and its elaboration of domestic detail" (Gilbert 2014, 148), but also by more sweeping cultural changes: "as a genre the culinary memoir was framed and informed by the increasing popularity of the cookbook in the ever more servantless twentieth century, along with the concomitant growth of mass cultural modes of personal and household instruction, including how-to books, food polemics, self-help diets, and even testimonial advertising" (Gilbert 2014, 148).

The popularity of food writing in France, however, as Ferguson explains in *Word of Mouth*, was a different story. In ways that were set up earlier by the French revolution and issues of starvation and class consciousness, the nineteenth century in France marked the beginning of an enormously popular trend toward the discussion of food at all levels: hence, there "emerge[d] a consciousness of food writing as a distinct genre born in response to the conditions of contemporary society. For some, food became a social issue; for others, a fashion; and for still others, a lens through which to examine and imagine the new world coming into being around them" (Ferguson 2014, 52–53). Jean Anthelme Brillat-Savarin, whose aphorisms about food are still quoted today ("you are what you eat" evolved out of his words, "dis-moi ce que tu manges, je te dirai ce que tu es"), and whose book *The Physiology of Taste* was published in 1826, was hugely influential; as Ferguson says, "it is Brillat whom we read and reread, quote and remember" (Ferguson 2014, 66).

Contemporary thinkers about food seem to agree, though, that we wouldn't have the kinds of food writing that we have today without the luminous presence of M.F.K. Fisher, whose musings on cuisine in many volumes, collected in 1990 in *The Art of Eating*, exerted a major influence on the genre. Gilbert, for instance, lauds *The Gastronomical Me* as "arguably the paradigmatic twentieth-century work of this sort . . . primarily a coming-of-age story . . . but . . . also a cultural history, a culinary polemic, a first-person tale of love and death—and thus a grief memoir—and even an informal cookbook" (Gilbert 2014, 144). It's hard to find someone who writes passionately about food who doesn't cite Fisher as having a significant impact.

Fisher was an American writer based in California who spent her formative years in France, and who introduced a new type of food writing when her books like *Serve It Forth* (1937), *Consider the Oyster* (1941), *How to Cook a Wolf* (1942), *The Gastronomical Me* (1943), and *An Alphabet for Gourmets* (1949) began to appear. Her work was innovative, and hugely influential for later food writers (especially the women memoirists whose work I will consider in chapter 7 of this volume), for several reasons. As I'll discuss, she practiced a certain level of class snobbery and her outlook at times was not necessarily what we would now consider feminist. But her *oeuvre* is significant on several counts. She was an original in her willingness to incorporate, in ways that were actually rather shocking at the time, her personal stories with her accounts of meals and her recipes. She was irreverent about others' normative beliefs about what to eat, when, how, and where. And her attention to hunger, pleasure, and sensuality—none of which were "appropriate" topics for a genteel woman to write about—was lyrical and self-disclosing in unprecedented ways.

It seems to have made a difference that Fisher's childhood did not allow her much room for thinking about food in pleasant ways. As she recounts, she was raised by a grandmother who forbade pleasure in eating or talk about food at the dinner table. Gilbert goes so far as to link Fisher's early food experiences to the development of a narrative style that bordered on a kind of brinksmanship:

> Fisher's portrait of her childhood cuisine as sometimes problematic— from the strictures of an ascetic grandmother to the deeds of a mad cook to the unpleasant experiments of a feckless schoolgirl—is central to her culinary-literary enterprise at its most successful. For whether as public performance or private experience, dining is always a source of some danger as well as carefully cultivated delight in this writer's imaginative world. And for these reasons it is often associated, as well, with both eroticism and gamesmanship. (Gilbert 2014, 155)

As an example, Gilbert calls attention to a particularly provocative episode in *The Gastronomical Me* in which Fisher, in rather openly erotic terms, describes her girlhood experience of a kind of sexual initiation when she is the object of desire for two different girls at her boarding school dance and ends up tasting her first oyster.

Fisher hated it that the Americans of the era (late 1930s–1940s) were so "ungastronomic" (Ferguson 2014, 100). She felt contempt for those whom she deemed incapable of taste, and as Megan Elias says, she made this contempt "bitingly clear" (Elias 2017, 77). In her efforts to distance herself from what she saw as the overly feminine eating habits of the time, she "emphasized," as Elias adds, "at every opportunity that she was not like other women" (Elias 2017, 102), even at times assuming a masculinist imperative in her food behavior and her narratives about it. When she laments the typical American hors-d'oeuvres of the time, for instance—the tray of small, fussy canapés—she cries, "What emasculation they have undergone, these pretty and miniscular appetizers!" (Fisher 1949, 195–96). Her famous wartime era ode to living well despite rationing and despair, *How to Cook a Wolf*, is aimed in a certain way at a feminine audience, with advice on how to look pretty in the kitchen and not get onion fumes in one's hair; she suggests keeping a mirror nearby with a little shelf for a lipstick and compact in case unexpected guests show up.

Yet much of her gender positioning is tongue-in-cheek, as if she is both playing into the expectations of feminine roles and subverting them at the same time; she never fails to suggest that she is the one who holds the power. Her recipe in *An Alphabet for Gourmets* for how to "unseduce" a man makes this clear. She says, "A wanton woman who could knowingly lead a man toward bed might just as easily, according to my talkative advisers, turn him away from it; and perhaps a whole dictionary of non-love should be written, about how to prepare this and that food most sure to stem desire" (Fisher 1949, 172). Fisher goes on to describe just such a meal, beginning with three Martinis and continuing with copious amounts of liquor and rich foods—"I would waste no time on a salad," she says, and the dessert "would be cold, superficially refreshing and tempting, but venomous: a chilled bowl of figs soaked in kirsch, with heavy cream" (Fisher 1949, 172–73). Of course, the phrase "according to my talkative advisers" is spurious: Fisher herself is in command of the knowledge here, but she feels somewhat winkingly obligated to pretend that she is merely passing on information that others have shared with her. More than that, she reveals how the cook, a woman, can wield tremendous power through the ability to seduce and "unseduce" at will, and through the narrative equivalent of the unseduction itself: the description of the meal sounds sensual, yet she uses it playfully to imply that there is a kind of witchcraft (the use of the word "venomous") involved in a kind of sexual manipulation through food. At the end of this little narrative, with no small degree of self-satisfaction, she remarks, "All of this would be beautiful fare in itself and in another part of time and space. Here and now it would be pure poison—given the right man. I would, to put it mildly, rest inviolate. What a hideous plan!" (Fisher 1949,

173). In other words, despite the playful reference to old-world values of chastity and maidenhood ("rest inviolate"), she's clearly asserting that she is the one in control: not just of the menu, but also of the narrative.

There's a lot more to be said about this issue of gender and power in Fisher's work, and many others have looked at this and other themes via the subtly revealed details of her autobiography. For my purposes here, I'm especially interested in how she talks about hunger in its literal and metaphorical manifestations. The way she interweaves the different forms that hunger can take exemplifies how food writing is always about more than just food, and "close-reading" a few of these moments demonstrates part of my approach to the works I discuss in the chapters that follow.

As mentioned earlier, *How to Cook a Wolf* was a wartime exercise in creating hope at a time of despair, and a rather idiosyncratic how-to book about the need for acting civilized in the midst of desperately barbarous behaviors—and doing so through food in a time when it was not plentiful. The original version of the book ends with a recipe for "Fruits aux Sept Liqueurs"—quite an escapist dish—to which she adds the remark, "Yes, it is crazy, to sit savoring such impossibilities, while headlines yell at you and the wolf whuffs through the keyhole" (Fisher 1942, 198). But then, in a conclusion that Fisher added to the volume later, she says that while she only knows a couple of gluttons who live to eat, she knows of countless others who would be better off if they "bent their spirits to the study of their own hungers" (Fisher 1942, 199). She claims that "[t]here are too many of us . . . who feel an impatience for the demands of our bodies, and who try throughout our whole lives, none too successfully, to deafen ourselves to the voice of our various hungers" (Fisher 1942, 199). While some, she says, try to do this through religion and some through a denial of sexual pleasure, she believes that there is a "dignity" one can find "in the face of poverty and war's fears and pains" by "nourish[ing] ourselves with all possible skill, delicacy, and ever-increasing enjoyment" (Fisher 1942, 200). It's an interesting afterword, as she seems to have realized that her audience may have taken issue with the very idea of a book about dining well published at a time when there were far greater concerns on the horizon. Yet what she is saying here is that hunger is not only about more than appetite: acknowledging it in its various connected forms is central to upholding our civilization. It's a grand claim, but it allows us to see how her thinking about food was not merely an exercise in narcissism.

She defends herself further in the often-quoted Foreword to *The Gastronomical Me*, wherein she responds to people who ask her why she chooses to write about food instead of "the struggle for power and security, and about love, the way others do" (Fisher 1943, ix). The obvious answer is that in writing about food, she really is writing about those other issues. Her response, though, is more complex, as it focuses, again, on the theme of hunger:

> The easiest answer is to say that, like most other humans, I am hungry. But there is more than that. It seems to me that our three basic needs, for food and security and love, are so mixed and mingled and intertwined that we cannot straightly think of one without the others. So it happens that when I write of hunger, I am really writing about love and the hunger for it, and warmth and the love of it and the hunger for it . . . and then the warmth and richness and fine reality of hunger satisfied . . . and it is all one. (Fisher 1943, ix; ellipses in original)

After she acknowledges the inseparability of different kinds of hungers, she "performs" this, in a sense, in her prose in the sentence that begins "So it happens." by deliberately getting lost in the repetitions of love/hunger/warmth and by using the ellipses to suggest both infinite repetition and the act of getting lost in her own reverie. There's a kind of immersiveness here that speaks to her awareness of how words, too, can be taken in, consumed, digested, and form some sort of nourishment or sensual solace.

She continues this theme in her Foreword to *An Alphabet for Gourmets* when she admonishes that "it is futile to consider hunger as a thing separate from people who are hungry" (Fisher 1949, ix). Indeed, she says, "If a woman can be made more peaceful, a man fuller and richer, children happier, by a changed approach to the basically brutish satisfaction of hunger, why should not I, the person who brought about that change, feel a definite and rewarding urge to proselytize?" (Fisher 1949, ix–x). The gender terms are, as always, a bit unsettling here: saying that a woman needs to be made "more peaceful" is perhaps a subtle dig at those who would claim that women—implicitly or especially her—are seen as hysterical troublemakers who require calming. She couches her response in the form of a rhetorical question, as if she is pretending to require permission to move forward, and yet she doesn't shy away from the somewhat self-mocking idea that her ultimate aim is to "proselytize," therefore also appropriating a religious term for the purposes of talking about food—and this is also another gender performance, since preaching would have more typically been a male rhetorical position. She even takes it a step further by underscoring that this proselytizing comes from a "definite and rewarding urge," therefore not shying away from an ownership of definitiveness, a pleasure in getting what one is owed, and above all in the decidedly (for the time) unfeminine admission of an "urge"—a yearning, a hunger.

Later in *An Alphabet for Gourmets*, she considers the twinned themes of hunger and gluttony, and this is also where she becomes more directly self-revelatory about the interplay between her own hungers or cravings and the extent to which she is willing to satisfy them. She admits that at present, especially compared to when she was younger, she isn't much of a glutton: "It is true that I overeat at times, through carelessness or a deliberate prolonging of my pleasure in a certain taste . . . [but now] I am probably incapable, really, of such lust. I rather regret it: one more admission of my dwindling powers!" (Fisher 1949, 49). She then adds that she's probably only really gluttonous when she has a wonderful bottle of wine in front of her: "I think to myself, when again will I have this taste upon my tongue?" (Fisher 1949, 49). The connection here between eating and sexual/orgasmic pleasure is obvious, especially as the two coalesce with her use of the word "lust" to denote the hunger for (ostensibly) food. And as always, she's playing with her readers, immediately following her pretended lament for her "dwindling powers" with a kind of braggadocio about her ability to down a whole bottle of wine at one sitting—in itself mitigated by the lyrical, Keatsian insistence on taking joy in the moment: "Where else in the world is there just such wine as this, with just this bouquet, at just this heat, in just this crystal cup?" (Fisher 1949, 49–50).

In "From A to Z: The Perfect Dinner," the closing chapter of *An Alphabet for Gourmets*, Fisher elaborates upon what she might eat if she were dining alone in the wintertime. The passage is as illuminating in terms of *how* she goes about satisfying her hunger as it is in terms of what she chooses to eat:

> I drink some *good* vermouth . . . and eat a little thinly sliced smoked salmon (this is a dream, of course, winter or summer), and then a completely personal and capricious concoction, shrimps or lobster tails or chicken in a thin, artful sauce, very subtle indeed, the kind that I like to pretend would be loathed by anyone but me. I eat it with a spoon and fork. I have a piece of good toast at hand, but I hardly touch it. And I sip, from a large, lone Swedish goblet, all its mates being long since shattered, a half-bottle of well-chilled fairly dry white wine; there is something delicately willful and decadent about drinking all alone no matter how small the bottle. And then, after one ruminative look at the little zabaglione I have painstakingly made for myself sometime earlier that day (I enjoy desserts in theory, but seldom can come to the actuality of eating them), I close the refrigerator door firmly upon it and go to bed, bolstered by books to be read and a hundred unattended dreams to be dreamed. (Fisher 1949, 213)

This passage, without ever mentioning the word "hunger," tells us quite a bit about Fisher's attitude toward eating and the art of self-satisfaction. Her description is shot through with an emphasis on singularity, from the *good* (italics Fisher's) vermouth to the idea of the main course as "personal and capricious" to the one remaining glass whose "mates" have been "shattered": in other words, the meal itself is about one-ness. The description is framed by the images of dreaming, from the "this is a dream, of course" to the ending phrase about going to bed with "dreams to be dreamed": in this sense, there is something phantasmagorical about the whole reverie. Her defiance at being judged is paralleled with a refusal to be judged, as she claims—or, importantly, "like[s] to pretend" that others would "loathe" her main course and that her drinking the wine alone is "delicately willful and decadent," and yet there is clearly no small measure of pride in these assertions. Perhaps most interesting here, though, is her treatment of the dessert course. The dessert that she made is "little," thus underlining the fact that she dared to make it only for herself and for no one else: she was not trying to please a man or any other diner. The look that she gives it before deciding not to eat it is "ruminative," meaning that she has given it fair consideration, as if in communion with it, showing that it is food for thought or that food is worthy of thought. But this is also an act of deferral, as she tells us about it but decides *not* to eat it. On the one hand, she put a lot of effort into making it ("painstakingly"); on the other hand, she seems to satisfy her hunger for it merely by studying it briefly in the refrigerator, as if to say that simply the act of having prepared it, possessing it, and (as is the case for us as readers) describing it as being present (with all of the lusciousness that a zabaglione entails) is, in the end, quite enough.

ON (NOT) FOLLOWING THE RECIPE

What can we learn about recipes from their narrative form, and what can we learn about narrative form itself from reading recipes? At its most basic level, a recipe is a formula, a set of instructions. Cookbooks are what Megan Elias calls "aspirational texts": "Sometimes we aspire to make just one recipe; at other times we more broadly reach for the lifestyle and values presented in a book" (Elias 2017, 4). And yet a recipe is always, almost by definition, a faulty approximation of a dish. It may surprise some people to learn that even in restaurant kitchens, cooks don't follow recipes exactly; when they create a stock, for example, they use what they have on hand. As Gary A. Fine says in his study *Kitchens: The Culture of Restaurant Work*, "Although cooks have recipes, they ignore them, interpret them, and move beyond them to creative autonomy" (Fine 1996, 24). He adds, "The evanescent character of cooking, distinguishing it from most other arts that are either material or can be captured in a written, auditory, or visual record, allows for imprecision that is not possible elsewhere" (Fine 1996, 26). One might see cooking as akin to a dance or theater performance, then, in the sense that like a performance, no completed dish—due to variations in measurements, plating, ingredient choices, temporal and weather factors, and even the mood or caprices of the cook—is ever exactly the same each time. And so almost by definition, a recipe is a narrative in flux, a mediated entity, a promise rather than the fulfillment of a promise.

The idea of a recipe has been embodied in cliché ("that's a recipe for disaster") and poets have used the recipe format for non-recipe topics; recipes have been incorporated into works of fiction (see Ntozake Shange's *Sassafrass, Cypress & Indigo*, or the over-the-top magical realist [and yet mostly makeable] recipes in Laura Esquivel's *Like Water for Chocolate*). As Sandra Gilbert says, "[t]here are recipes for poisons, recipes for witches' brews, recipes for revenge and recipes shot through with grief," citing Patricia Smith's stunning recipe-format poem about her father, "When the Burning Begins," as one example (Gilbert 2014, 296–97). More often than not, food memoirs—including most of the ones discussed later in this volume—include recipes, sometimes in disconcerting form. Recipes are personal: they tell us something about ourselves. Gilbert remarks, "Our recipes are histories of who we are, transmitting the tastes of the past through precept and example, even as they suggest how we can sometimes revise our lives by adjusting the menu" (Gilbert 2014, 8).

Beyond that, adding recipes gives the writer's narrative a certain kind of legitimacy—if this is a food memoir, then the author needs to be able to show in some more concrete way than just the narrative portions that (s)he possesses a certain level of expertise. But they also thus engage us in a different kind of reading experience than we would have if we were only reading regular paragraphs. Including recipes allows food memoirists to engage the reader's senses and palate in a more overt way; it provides the chance to move spatially or temporally to a different point in the narrative; and it challenges genre boundaries by requiring, quite simply, that we direct (or fail to direct) our attention to an alternative type of readerly interpretation.

We don't tend to read a recipe the same way we read a piece of prose. If we are intending to make the dish, we skim it once to see whether we have the ingredients on hand (or we forget to do so, and have to make a last-minute substitution or abandon the dish altogether). We skim it again to find out whether the oven has to be preheated, what kind of dishes or pans we need, and how many servings the recipe makes. And then we read through it more carefully a third time, but this reading is interrupted by the physical steps involved in preparing the dish. Sometimes, after we have finished making a dish, we annotate the recipe with thoughts about how it tasted, when/where we served it, whether we would make it again, and what we did or would do differently—and so we also become editors or new authors of the recipe's narrative. And yet, reading a recipe feels somehow out of place or—for some readers—uninteresting in the context of another style of narrative as opposed to when these readers are actively seeking something to prepare; every time I ask my students, when we're reading a food memoir, whether they actually read the included recipes, they admit to just having skimmed over them, except for any parts that offer irreverent or surprising advice that seems pertinent to the theme of the memoir itself. Including something as mundane as a recipe in a high-culture piece of writing about food was initially a daring act. M.F.K. Fisher did so a bit hesitantly, saying that if recipes are to appear in her work, they will be "like birds in a tree—if there is a comfortable branch" (Fisher 1990, 6).

Commonly, today, if you need a recipe for something, you might go to a site like epicurious.com to find it, or you might look through your collection of cookbooks or cooking magazines. Some of us have file boxes or scrapbooks with beloved family recipes that a parent, aunt or uncle, or grandparent wrote down—or that we tried to write down ourselves when said relative refused to share one and insisted that it's just something you learn by watching. Or that we regret never having even tried to write down. To this day, my sisters and I have tried countless times to duplicate our late grandma's indescribably sublime brisket, and we have come close, but since we never found out how she made it, the secrets have been lost: did she add tomato sauce? Carrots? Wine? How long did she keep it in the oven? We'll never know for sure. Stephen Steinberg asks similar questions in his essay about his grandmother's challah bread and the idea that no one of the next two generations has ever been able to duplicate it; he goes so far as to wonder whether this was on some level even a deliberate act, out of a kind of denial of mortality:

> Perhaps the answer is obvious: that we all conspired in the comfortable illusion that my grandmother and her challah would be here forever. Perhaps we wished to remain children, which was possible so long as we were fed by the family matriarch. Perhaps we realized, on some level of consciousness, that my grandmother's challah would not be the same if the dough were not kneaded by *her* hands, if it were not baked in *her* oven, and if it were not purveyed by *her* outstretched arms, accompanied by her loving embrace. Perhaps it was right that the secret should remain hers, not to be simulated by some pretender. But then again, how was culture ever purveyed from one generation to the next? (Steinberg 1998, 296)

A recipe, then, might be about a legacy or about the anxiety over or the lack of a legacy. As I discuss later in this book, the women in the concentration camp in Terezín, as they were starving, stayed up late at night and traded (even argued over) recipes for elaborate pastries and other dishes for which they had no access to the ingredients: they found comfort in formulas and measurements, and they survived in part (or a handful did) by using the narrative form of the recipe as an alternative to food itself, as a source of sustenance and hope. Reading a recipe requires an imagination, a visualization of how a dish would come together and how it would taste, and an imagination was required for these women to have any sense of optimism that they would survive.

In a certain way, a recipe is a palimpsest, a text that has been written and rewritten with traces of its previous writing (which we sometimes see, in older/annotated recipes). Even a recipe in a cookbook or cooking magazine has presumably been tested and rewritten numerous times. And the cookbooks that we use most often are more than likely smudged with food. Megan J. Elias begins her study of cookbooks, *Food on the Page*, with an amusing attention to the idea of recipes that have marks, notes, and food stains:

> I once bought a secondhand copy of a Fannie Farmer Cookbook in which a previous reader had written and underlined the word "no" next to a recipe for soft custard. I myself have since made clear my allegiance to a particular chocolate pudding recipe through spine wear as I opened the book to it many times and through glops of batter dropped on the page, expressing my own version of "yes." The little direct evidence of cooking that occurs in physical cookbooks comes in the form of such personal annotations and stains. (Elias 2017, 1)

Even online, when users of a site like epicurious.com prepare a recipe, they might return to it and offer notes in the commentary section about substitutions that they made or about the success (or lack thereof) of the finished dish.

And a cookbook, more often than not, is much more than just a set of instructions. Elias's study points out that the earliest American cookbooks (going back to 1796) were "prescriptive" in a manner that continued through most of the 1800s: "the collections of recipes and household guidance that were the norm through most of the nineteenth century . . . forcefully claimed their authors' knowledge and readers' ignorance" (Elias 2017, 4). As Henry Notaker points out in his gloriously detailed history of the genre, "A cookbook is basically a collection of recipes for the preparation of food. But cookbooks contained a mix of recipes, household advice, cultural background information, anecdotes, reminiscences, and personal commentaries since long before the advent of printing" (Notaker 2017, x). Notaker also reminds us that the cook(s) who create a recipe may be, but are not necessarily, the same people as the writer(s) who put them into cookbook form. In fact, his description of how these two roles would have often been separated in earlier years helps us to understand in a larger way that the narrative of a recipe is complicated by a kind of triangular relationship:

> [T]he writer who records the recipe, if he is not documenting it only as a personal aide-memoire, must position himself in relation to another addressee, not a pupil or a daughter by his or her side, but rather a reader or readers, who are invisible to the writer. Therefore, the writer must bring into the recipe all the things and acts a pupil would be able to observe directly but that cannot be seen by the reader, such as utensils, actions, and the physical actions necessary to handle them. (Notaker 2017, 55)

When we create a recipe, we are trying for an approximation of a moment of deliciousness, but that moment may have relatively little to do with the recipe itself. A recipe always by necessity falls short of the actual replication and consumption of a dish that was perfect in a given moment in the past. We can't get the past back again, but we can, like Proust, capture its essence for a moment in the act of smelling or tasting food. In *Life without a Recipe*—a memoir whose title itself speaks to the nature of improvisation—Diana Abu-Jaber beautifully describes the way in which a recipe somehow tends to fall short of what we actually want or remember:

> Most dishes aren't written down. They hover in the memory, a bit of contrail, the ends uncertain. What lingers are the traces, the way the vanilla dallied with the ginger, fading from the tongue like a last thread of salt. The taste, as it's remembered and passed down, can rarely be duplicated; the steps are mislaid, the ingredients tampered with. The taste is desire itself, the yearning for completion, in love or sugar or blood. Each recipe is someone else's mistake or discovery. (Abu-Jaber 2016, 41)

In *The Outlaw Cook*, John Thorne decries gadgets like the food processor and the microwave for having estranged us from real, time-intensive, hands-on connections to the foods that we are making. He argues, too, against recipes, claiming that their predetermined ingredients and measurements run counter to the idea in many culinary traditions (such as Italian) that the cook should re-create what (s)he is preparing each time according to what (s)he has on hand, what the demands are of those about to eat the meal, and so forth. Thorne further claims that the impersonal nature of most recipes fails to take into account the actual "needs or appetites" of the diners themselves:

> There is something relentless about recipes in this regard: they create a condition not unlike the air temperature in a large office building, where it is always too hot in the winter and too cold in the summer— but if no one is really happy, neither can anyone complain. Recipe cooking likewise gives us too much; whether in the guise of fattening us up or slimming us down, somehow things are always being waved in front of our mouths. This is the purpose of recipes, after all: to arouse appetite. Like central heating, food writing's only task is to make us "comfortable": it might be establishing a climate of self-indulgence or self-denial, but it is still busy making us feel hungry—the only question being what we are to become hungry *for*. (Thorne 2015, 284)

While Thorne has a point about how there is sometimes an oddly dictatorial element to recipes, his argument is perhaps too rigid if we consider that food writers—in memoirs, and sometimes even in magazines like *Food & Wine* or *Bon Appétit*—also have played deliberately against the seeming inflexibility or tedium of the form. His emphasis on the constant appeal to us to eat, the relentless display of food or its preparation or consumption, is certainly applicable in the world of the Food Network and Instagram. But as a written narrative, there's more room for free play in the recipe format than Thorne might have us believe. Part of the pleasure of unconventional food writing, particularly as memoirists (or fiction writers like Esquivel) embed recipes into their stories, is that the authors play deliberately with language that is seemingly excessive, inappropriately personal, irrelevant, or even not especially appetizing. The recipe may be included more to make a point—as Sandra Gilbert does in reference to communities, food, and grieving families when she gives the one for the "American Legion Funeral Hot Dish," which includes a lot of frozen vegetables, a bag of chow mein noodles, and two kids of condensed soup (Gilbert 2014, 42)—than to provide us with instructions for something we would actually want to make or eat. If we're about to skim over one of these recipes, we might do a double-take when we see how it is written. Sometimes the intention is still to make us hungry, but sometimes the recipe expresses such a deeply felt memory or anxiety that its telling is not really at all about the dish itself.

Many of the food memoirists whose works I will discuss later in this volume play, sometimes wistfully or nostalgically, sometimes sarcastically, with the recipe form, at times even mocking the genre itself. In Julie Powell's *Cleaving*—her sequel to *Julie and Julia*, which I talk about in this book—she provides a recipe for her husband Eric's pork chops, yet her narrative of the recipe seems to be, rather entertainingly, at odds with itself. At the beginning of the recipe, she tells us to heat the vegetable oil until it is "almost smoking," then adds the following parenthetical comment:

> (Don't you love it when recipes say things like "almost smoking"? Reminds me of that Beckett story about a stage direction reading that a door should be "imperceptibly ajar." Fuck you, Beckett. The oil can be smoking a little. Or not. Just make sure it's good and hot.) (Powell 2009, 38)

There are a couple of things going on here. In the context of the memoir, Powell—whose marriage to Eric is in a growing state of crisis as the book continues and she is simultaneously involved in an extramarital affair and is learning to become a butcher—is playing out her newfound fascination with meat after she has just brought the Berkshire pork chops home and says that she "prattle[s] on" about it and is "a little manic" (Powell 2009, 39). Meat, in this memoir, is intimately connected with her efforts to understand sexuality and attachment or cutting away. But her Beckett reference—especially with the "Fuck you, Beckett"—reflects a willful and playful arrogance that in some ways masks a larger set of insecurities; she parallels the rejection of the conventional recipe instruction phrase with the rejection of a high-culture playwright, and yet she's showing off a bit here by invoking Beckett in the first place—in the middle of a simple recipe, of all things—as if to say that she actually knows how to make pork chops in a fancier way but that she also at this point in the memoir wants to acknowledge her husband's cooking (as long as she gets to create the recipe's narrative in her own terms).

Adam Gopnik, in a brilliant 2009 essay originally published in *The New Yorker* called "What's the Recipe? Our Hunger for Cookbooks," takes on the question of why we turn to recipes when they are always, on some level, an exercise in frustration. He says, "Anyone who cooks knows that it is in following recipes that one first learns the anticlimax of the actual, the perpetual disappointment of the thing achieved" (Gopnik 2015, 457). He describes the way that recipes attract us with their words' ability to instill in us a sense of longing or an enjoyment of the steps involved in the act of creation, and yet to frustrate us with the difficulty of understanding how exactly to interpret their meaning. In a manner that reflects Powell's frustration with the term "almost smoking," he asks, "How do you know when a thing 'just begins to boil'? How can you be sure that milk has scorched but not burned? Or touch something too hot to touch, or tell firm peaks from stiff peaks?" (Gopnik 2015, 458). He concludes that even though the narrative of a recipe implies a level of confidence on the part of the narrator, the real secret is that there's often an "immense" gap between what the narrator tells us and what we're able to do (Gopnik 2015, 458).

As a result, he claims, cookbooks themselves have changed so that we read them perhaps less for the purpose of acquiring recipe information than for forging some kind of connection with the narrator (who is often a celebrity chef). The cookbook turns, he says, "like everything else these days, toward the memoir, the confessional, the recipe as self-revelation" (Gopnik 2015, 460). The paradox he invokes might remind us of the women of the Terezín concentration camp giving one another verbal versions of recipes to sustain themselves in the face of starvation: we read recipes despite the knowledge that they won't ever turn out quite the way we imagine them, and yet we keep reading because "the act of wanting ends up mattering more than the fact of getting" (Gopnik 2015, 464). Gopnik doesn't mention poststructuralist or psychoanalytical criticism—it's not appropriate for his readership, anyway—but what he is saying here embodies some of the same complex notions of pleasure and its deferment that we see writers like the two Jacques, Derrida and Lacan, considering in more theoretical context. Recipes provide a roadmap for the promise of gratification, its continual frustration, and the longing to create pleasure despite or even because of this frustration. And so we keep reading them (and perhaps buying colorful cookbooks), whether or not we intend to make the dishes therein. Elias's cookbook history points out that innovations in creating "cheaply print[ed] high-quality digital color photographs helped to increase the numbers and sizes of pictures in cookbooks and food magazines" (Elias 2017, 181); as the cookbook became "a thing of beauty," its "existence as a visual object frequently overshadowed its potential as an object of mechanical use" (Elias 2017, 182). As Notaker says about these beautiful coffee-table cookbooks that we perhaps don't even bring into the kitchen, their contents "are meant to be leafed through and read sitting in a sofa or an easy chair rather than followed step by step over the kitchen stove" (Notaker 2017, 301). The recipes, then, are displaced to the realm of the imagination.

OOOT BURGERS AND ONIONS

The recent scholarly interest in Object-Oriented Ontological Theory (also known as OOOT), though it sounds overly erudite, is of particular value when we think about the literature of food, and so it is worth a few short excursions into the OOOT world in order to understand how it might help us to "read" food as object and as text. This is not the right place for an elaborate explanation of what OOO theory is and how it works, so readers are referred to the seminal works in this area, such as Ian Bogost's *Alien Phenomenology*, Timothy Morton's *Realist Magic*, and Bill Brown's anthology *Things*, especially his introductory essay, "Thing Theory." In what follows, I will offer a capsule explanation of what OOOT is, followed by two ventures into OOOT analysis that may not be orthodox versions of this kind of theory (if there is such a thing), but that will demonstrate more specifically how it might be useful when we're considering food writing: let's examine the burger and then the onion.

To put it very briefly, OOO theorists believe that in our postmodern, possibly "posthuman" world, we might do more to consider things *as* things, to examine how objects not only take on a life of their own, but also how the deeply layered history of an object provides us with a wealth of cultural information, attention to the ways it changes and mutates over time, and a clearer understanding of how we, as humans, operate in relation to it when the object itself—rather than us—is given primary importance. Jane Bennett, in *Vibrant Matter*, credits French theorist Michel Foucault for legitimizing philosophical attention to bodily practices like eating. Paying attention to what she calls "thing-power" is important, she writes, as it "gestures toward the strange ability of ordinary, man-made items to exceed their status as objects and to manifest traces of independence or aliveness, constituting the outside of our own experience." Bennett's study includes a chapter on food in which, she says, "I present the case for edible matter as an actant operating inside and alongside humankind, exerting influence on moods, dispositions, and decisions" (Bennett 2010).

The plant or animal that gives us something to eat has or had a life of its own outside of our bodies. We cultivate, manufacture, purchase, prepare, consume, digest, and excrete it—all processes that involve complex interactions between us and it. To look at food through the lens of OOOT is to perform a new form of close-reading, and doing so can be highly entertaining and illuminating. When we focus uniquely on something in particular that we eat, whether it is an Oreo cookie or a plate of fettucine alfredo, we uncover an entire deep structure of it. We unpack the recipe; we scrutinize the ingredients; we look at the origins of the dish; we place it in its cultural milieu; we explore the ethics or value of consuming it; we therefore understand more fully how this food item has been created and transformed, even in ways beyond its original status or intentions. The small books in Bloomsbury's "Object Lessons" series have been especially useful examples of how to practice an OOOT-based exploration of a thing in its thingness; the series covers mostly non-food objects such as Golf Ball, Dust, Glass, Hotel, etc., but a few of these volumes take on items of food such as Bread or Egg, while others, such as Refrigerator, are food-related. Meditating closely on one item that we eat is something that food writers have done for a long time, but such a practice was never really validated in the critical establishment until OOO, heavily influenced by the earlier Continental philosophical practice of phenomenology (e.g., Husserl and others) and by Roland Barthes (*Mythologies*), reinforced the idea that an everyday object (as opposed to an abstract concept) has profound layers of meaning.

Carol Adams's recent contribution to the Object Lessons series, *Burger*, illustrates what this kind of reading can do. Adams is well known as a feminist writer who advocates for consciousness-raising about the implications of eating meat; her book *The Sexual Politics of Meat* is discussed in my consideration of food and performance art in chapter 5. She's an unusual and perhaps controversial choice for the Burger subject, since she does not eat meat herself and does not spend time describing or celebrating the taste of a really superb hamburger, except for twice when she taste-tests a vegetarian burger in development. However, the book demonstrates the wide range of material that surrounds the creation, distribution, and consumption of the burger, such that if you read it, you'll never look at an ordinary McDonald's hamburger in the same way again.

Her study contains many references to the work of Eric Schlosser (*Fast Food Nation*), Michael Pollan, and others who have written celebrated explanations of the real (and alarmingly gruesome) story behind how cattle are made into burgers, as well as a cultural history of the development of hamburger franchises by Ray Kroc and others; she looks at disturbing recent ad campaigns that "make" women into hamburgers; and she fast-forwards to scientists who are attempting to replicate the smell and taste of a burger with plant-based and synthetic ingredients. In all of this, though, she undertakes a more precise project: in a sense, she lifts the bun off of the burger, asks us to put our eyes, nose, and tongue close to it, and requires us to see it not just as the object in front of us but also as something that required a complex story in order to arrive on our plate. Adams asks:

> Has not the hamburger always been a sign of instability, around which superstructures (golden arches, castle turrets) are built in attempts to stabilize it, mythologize it? In *Reification, or The Anxiety of Late Capitalism*, Timothy Bewes suggests that reification contains within it its own resistance. Does the hamburger, that ultimate symbol of reification — thingifying living beings by shaping their dead bodies into meat — contain the making of its own dissolution/disappearance within it? And not only because dead bodies decay? Is the hamburger a modernist aberration, albeit a very successful one, in the long tradition of shaping protein food items into single-portion meals? If so, what is replacing it? The everyday object of burgerness. The non-meat burger is no longer the uncanny, the unbelievable. (Adams 2018, 135)

Clearly, Adams has an agenda here that not all readers will agree with — many of us probably wouldn't eat and enjoy meat if we weren't capable of fairly complex processes of denial about what we are doing — but her approach is a fascinating example of how we can use OOOT to "read" what is on our plate.

I may be more inclined to "read" the hamburger in front of me through a different set of potential narratives — how does this differ from or resemble other hamburgers I have eaten before? If it is a fast-food hamburger, am I relying on a kind of uniformity or sameness for reassurance? Am I eating this hamburger because I am genuinely hungry for it, to satisfy some kind of nostalgic or emotional hunger, or simply because I participated in the ritual of ordering food at a prescribed time? Do I like it because I like the hamburger itself, or because it is a vehicle for accoutrements I crave like ketchup and pickles? All of this involves a kind of mindfulness for which we usually don't have the time or the inclination, but Adams asks us to take this mindfulness a step further and to ask harder questions as well, about the origins and provenance of the burger and the ethical and ecological issues connected to its consumption. She might be accused of taking the joy out of the process of eating something pleasurable, but I would respond that there is another kind of pleasure in this kind of close attention, akin to the pleasure of close-reading a literary text: we might not like everything we learn or that the text evokes, but our world is expanded by our having paid more attention to it.

Another fascinating example of what might be called an OOOT food reading, although it is in no way labeled as such, is Robert Farrar Capon's consideration of the onion in his book *The Supper of the Lamb*. Capon was an Episcopal priest who also wrote food columns for publications like the *New York Times* and *Newsday*. Although some readers may be put off by the admittedly spiritual (and sometimes a bit wacky) viewpoint he has when he contemplates something like the onion, his meditation on it is

not only a beautiful piece of writing, but it shows — in a very, very different manner than Adams, whose OOOT reading in *Burger* was invested
primarily in the sociocultural/ecological implications of her food object —
what can transpire when we read (something on) a plate through its
status as a thing that has a life in relation to us, but also outside of us.

If an onion seems to be an overly mundane choice for lengthy consideration, that is precisely the point. No doubt Capon chooses the onion in
part because it is humble in nature, used everywhere, but also maligned
for its lingering scent and for the ability of its fumes to make people cry.
He begins by telling us that in order to appropriately contemplate the
onion, we shouldn't rush into peeling or cutting it; rather, we need to
plan on first spending an hour or so simply studying it, taking it in,
literally appreciating its layers of meaning. He knows that this sounds
like a rather ludicrous idea, and so, as he does throughout the piece, he
offers encouragement to the reader: "Admittedly, spending an hour in
the society of an onion may be something you have never done before.
You feel, perhaps, a certain resistance to the project. Please don't" (Capon
2015, 204–5).

As he asks us to look at and study the onion, his words embody
exactly what OOO theorists want us to consider as well: "You will note,
to begin with, that the onion is a *thing*, a being, just as you are" (Capon
2015, 205). His abstractions from this go in a more theological direction,
as he argues that by getting us in this moment to experience a sense of
place, we understand more deeply that what being in a place feels like is
not bound to time/space coordinates, and therefore we can better appreciate (through our meeting with the onion) what it is like to be aware of
an abstract place like heaven.

After we have communed at length with the onion, looking at it in a
way that we have never done before, he asks us to begin peeling its skin
off gently and to notice the skin's astounding dryness, marking how
"elegant" and "deliberate" that dryness is: "[d]ryness as an achievement,
not as a failure" (Capon 2015, 206). He then offers us a particularly revelatory moment as he points out that when we lay out the onion skin and
begin to look at the onion itself, we are in effect seeing something that no
one else has ever seen before — in other words, we are the only ones who
have seen inside this particular onion. Again, his interpretation has a
religious spin to is, but it's also a rather moving way of helping us remember that when we address ourselves to a plant that we are about to
eat, it's worth appreciating its singular and secret status: the onion layers
"present themselves to you as the animals to Adam: as nameless till seen
by man . . . They come as deputies of all the hiddennesses of the world, of
all the silent competencies endlessly at work deep down things" (Capon
2015, 207).

The next step, he tells us, is to cut the onion, and thus to become
aware of its inner life: not only its colors, but when we press upon it, its

moisture. Although his language to describe this is again hyperbolic, this time intimating not only the religious but also a kind of primal childbirth image—"the sea within all life has tipped its hand"—his characterization is illuminating because it again forces us to acknowledge the independent thing-ness of the onion. He writes, "You have cut open no inanimate thing, but a living tumescent being" (Capon 2015, 207), and demands that we consider "what a soul the onion must have, if it boasts such juices" (Capon 2015, 208). As he has us press upon the onion with our fingers so that it releases its juices upon them, he takes the opposite approach of the many who would explain how to get rid of the smell of onions on your hands, and exalts instead that "the onion is now part of you" and that "[i]t will be for days" as its scent lingers on your skin (Capon 2015, 209).

It's pretty clear here that the onion for Capon is perhaps a stand-in for a vagina, but it's also a form of transubstantiation. Whatever we think of his unabashedly over-the-top descriptions, his insistence that we pay attention to the moment's spiritual gravity, and his ultimate point that understanding the onion allows us to understand the mysteries of creation, we can take to heart his reminder that this little experiment (or reading about it) has helped us to see that "a thing is more than the sum of all the insubstantialities that comprise it" (Capon 2015, 209). This is an elegant way for those of us who care about food to appreciate how close-reading a food item (through the lens of OOOT, even when not patently acknowledged as such) brings us even closer to what we eat.

The structure of this volume takes the reader from representations of food in literary form (such as the poetry of Whitman and Ginsberg) to its less conventional manifestations in performance art to its importance in recent food memoirs. To be more specific, I move from a consideration of food in primarily literary genres (in chapters 2, 3, and 4) to a transitional section that treats performance art (which is both literary and extraliterary) and mixed-genre comparative cultural analysis (in chapters 5 and 6) to the creative nonfiction/food memoir genre (in chapters 7, 8, and 9). My selection of texts to be considered is in certain ways based as much on personal preference as on broad cultural representation: it was important to me that these works include food cultures that have interested me for many years (as represented in the choices of Jewish, Indian, African American, and Asian authors) and that gender, so deeply connected to the study of food (as represented in the chapters on performance art, women's food memoirs, and male midlife crisis food memoirs) also has a starring role. And as a longtime Beat Studies scholar, Allen Ginsberg (and his poetic ancestor Walt Whitman), with his fierce and defiant hungers, was always a starting point. It was of course impossible to include many other works, particularly food memoirs and recipe-based novels, that would have fit here as well, but I hope that my somewhat idiosyncratic choice of texts allows the reader to consider alternative texts using the same tools for analysis. In the summary that follows, I have high-lighted both the focal texts and the central issues for each chapter.

Chapter 1 is entitled "The Hungry Yawp: Eating and Orality in Whit-man and Ginsberg," and focuses on questions of appetite and transcen-dence in works by these two poets. I consider the question of what the attention to food means for Beat Generation writers, and I explore the interconnectedness of Whitman's and Ginsberg's work in this context. Ultimately, while appetite for Whitman is celebratory and is connected to larger images of desire, it takes on more of a contentious political aspect in Ginsberg's poems.

Chapter 2, "The Politics of Gluttony in Second-Generation Holocaust Literature," highlights the Holocaust cookbook *In Memory's Kitchen*, Art Spiegelman's "survivor's tale" *Maus*, Donald Margulies's play *The Model Apartment*, and several works by contemporary post-Holocaust poets. Holocaust survivors (and consequently, their children, who are seen as survivors in another sense), as the result of enforced starvation (or, for their offspring, stories about starvation), tend to take on a preoccupation with food through behaviors of both hoarding and gluttony. This chapter discusses, through these works, what it means to be the child of a Holo-caust survivor, and how this is reflected in the experiences of food and eating.

Chapter 3 is called "Chukla Bukla: Cooking, Bengali-Indian-Anglo-American Writers, and the Merging of Cultures." It treats Anita Desai's novel *Fasting, Feasting*, Jhumpa Lahiri's short stories in *Unaccustomed Earth*, and Shelby Silas's play *Calcutta Kosher*. In these works, experiences of food embody larger questions about multicultural identities, social class standing, maternal relationships, and religious (in the case of Silas's play, Jewish-Hindu) practices and affiliations.

Chapter 4, "Feeding the Audience: Food, Feminism, and Performance Art," explores works by a wide range of women performance artists, including Karen Finley, Carolee Schneeman, and Bonnie Sherk. Here, I interrogate the connections between the public performance of eating and acts of transgression. My exploration focuses on how these artists parody and subvert images of the female body as an object of consump-tion, and how their work politicizes the sometimes-vexed relationship between eating and femininity.

In chapter 5, "The Last Black Man's Fried Chicken: Soul Food, Memo-ry, and African American Culinary Writing," I bring together the food writing of the late Ntozake Shange, Suzan-Lori Parks's play *The Death of the Last Black Man in the Whole Entire World*, and Jeff Henderson's memoir *Cooked: My Journey from the Streets to the Stove*. Shange's and Henderson's culinary prose and Parks's avant-garde play might appear to have little in common, but all three pay close attention to "soul food" and its history and preparation. They express fascinatingly complicated attitudes about the legacy of "soul food," the stereotypes connected with it, and its relevance to their audiences' lives.

Chapter 6 marks the transition to the last section of the book and is entitled "Cooking Up a Storm: Recent Food Memoirs and the Angry Daughter." A surprisingly significant number of works reflect the chapter's theme and are discussed here: Ayun Halliday's *Dirty Sugar Cookies*, Julie Powell's *Julie and Julia*, Kim Sunée's *Trail of Crumbs*, Laura Schenone's *The Lost Ravioli Recipes of Hoboken*, Gabrielle Hamilton's *Blood, Bones, and Butter*, Kate Moses's *Cakewalk*, Diana Abu-Jaber's *The Language of Baklava* and *Life without a Recipe*, and Ruth Reichl's *Tender at the Bone* and *Comfort Me with Apples*. I attempt here to explain the prevalence of women's food memoirs in which the *mother*, rather than serving the clichéd function of the Betty Crockerish cooking inspiration, becomes the force *against* which these narrators take refuge by turning to the kitchen. I also consider what the implications are when a father or other male figure (as in Sunée and Abu-Jaber) takes on the traditionally maternal role of culinary mentor.

Chapter 7, which can be seen as a companion piece to the previous chapter, is called "Eat and Run: Food Writing, Masculinity, and the 'Male Midlife Crisis.'" I discuss Anthony Bourdain's *Kitchen Confidential* and other works of his, as well as Jonathan Reynolds's *Wrestling with Gravy*, Bob Spitz's *The Saucier's Apprentice*, Frank Bruni's *Born Round*, and Marcus Samuelsson's *Yes, Chef*. My emphasis here is on how being a son (instead of a daughter) influences these narrators' attitudes towards food and cooking. For these narrators, in later life, crises of sexuality, marriage/divorce, body image, and cultural identification affect their masculine identity positions and their subsequent attempts (with varying degrees of success) to create new subjectivities through food.

Chapter 8, "School Lunch: Bicultural Conflicts in Asian-American Women's Food Memoirs," concludes the textual explorations in this volume with a focus on Bich Minh Nguyen's *Stealing Buddha's Dinner* and Linda Furiya's *Bento Box in the Heartland*, and with a closing look at Ava Chin's foraging memoir *Eating Wildly*. Nguyen's and Furiya's memoirs use food to depict the struggle between identification with one's native culture and the childhood longing for assimilation into a normative American culture. In their Vietnamese-American (Nguyen) and Japanese-American (Furiya) households, secrecy and shame—but also anger and pride—factor into the narrators' developing "food lives." The "school lunch" in these (and other) works becomes a trope that exemplifies the conflicts that these narrators face. And Chin's book (rather literally) breaks new ground when it comes to integrating one's food past with the present.

The conclusion invokes two current trends in food literature not discussed in previous chapters: food journalism by writers like Eric Schlosser and Michael Pollan that urge us to be more aware of what is on our plates, and behind-the-scenes memoirs about restaurant work by Pete Jordan (*Dishwasher*) and others. I connect these trends to the book's larger purpose of close-reading, culminating in a discussion of an essay about ice cream that prompted a very specific food narrative of my own. And with the hope that the offerings promised in this volume sound appetizing, I invite the reader to join me at the table.

ONE

The Hungry Yawp

Eating and Orality in Whitman and Ginsberg

For the nineteenth-century American poet Walt Whitman as well as for many of the writers of the Beat Generation of the mid-1950s to the mid-1960s, eating is both a physically grounding and a transcendent act. It reminds the writer that the body *is* a body, with appetites and hungers, but it is also a marker of awareness of the metaphysical and spiritual worlds. I will argue in this chapter that while Whitman negotiates constantly between the earthy/sensual side of eating and its metaphorical aspects, eating for Beat poet Allen Ginsberg is politically charged, laden with the historical and poetic past.

The great food writer M.F.K. Fisher, whose work I discussed in the introduction to this volume, says in her Foreword to the 1949 classic *An Alphabet for Gourmets* that we can't separate hunger from the person who is hungry (Fisher 1949, ix–x). And yet when we talk about food or taste, finding a common language in which to do so is more difficult than one might imagine; as food philosopher Gary Alan Fine puts it in his study of "the aesthetics of kitchen discourse," the challenge is "to transform this individual experience into collective expression . . . Consuming pretzels, I cannot determine if your sensation of salty is identical to my sensation of salty" (Fine 1996, 217). And in what may be a fancy way of saying that we are what we eat, Deane Curtin's essay "Food/Body/Person" remarks, "To account for our openness to food requires a relational understanding of self" (Curtin 1992, 11). These three writers have very different points of view, but for all three, cooking or consuming food—or even talking about food with others—requires a kind of boundary-crossing, and this is the aspect of eating that particularly interests me in both Whitman's and Ginsberg's work.

I begin with the passage in which the speaker in "Song of Myself" depicts himself as: "Walt Whitman, a Kosmos, of Manhattan the son,/ Turbulent, fleshy, sensual,/eating, drinking and breeding" (Whitman 2004, 86). He later adds, "I believe in the flesh and the appetites" (Whitman 2004, 87) and is "[a]t apple-peelings wanting kisses for all the red fruit I find." And in "Song at Sunset," he exclaims, "To be conscious of my body, so satisfied, so large!" (Whitman 2004, 504). It goes almost without saying that Walt Whitman figures his poetic persona as a lover of the natural world, but the question remains of whether he is also a lover of food and drink—or, to be more prosaic about it, we might ask how and what Whitman eats in his poetry.

A similar question might be raised about several of the Beat Generation writers; scarcely a page of Jack Kerouac's *The Dharma Bums* goes by, for instance, without a specific and even obsessive attention to food. In 1961—a point at which Beat culture had become part of the broader pop culture (fostering TV shows like *Dobie Gillis*, *Mad* magazine parodies, and even Rent-a-Beatniks available for parties)—there was even a tongue-in-cheek *Beat Generation Cookbook* edited by Carl Larsen and James Singer. Its offerings included the Kerouac Kocktail and the Subterranean Spudnik, with the latter being touted as having been invented by a "young Beat doll who is also the mother of three Beatlets" (qtd. in Elias 2017, 156). Even though the cookbook was parodic, it provides some insights into what the Beats' attitude towards food and eating was perceived as being. Most of the recipes used the standard American pantry ingredients popular at the time, like canned soup, and most of them acknowledged the need for repurposing cheap ingredients, as we indeed witness in *The Dharma Bums*, or having to scrounge for food, as we see in Ginsberg's *Howl*. As Megan Elias suggests, the target for both the Beats and the cookbook itself was not the corruption of consumerist culture and the way we eat, but rather, the desire to forge something non-normative:

> The recipes served as a way to jest about American culture, in which contemporary cookbooks encouraged new mixtures of packaged goods. There was no identifiable cuisine at work aside from the haphazard, playing on the notion of the beatnik as improvisational. The beatnik scrounged his dinner from the supplies of mainstream culture instead of critiquing its palate or systems. (Elias 2017, 156)

That critique would come later, and even appeared, as we shall see, in Ginsberg's post-Beat era poems. What we see at play already here, though, is the difference between Whitman's sweeping declarations of love for the America of his time and experience, and the Beats' efforts to see post-World War II America from outside the mainstream, to reevaluate what is "holy," and perhaps to reinvent it. And yet, Whitman—in his sexuality, his poetic form, and his exuberance—had a profound influence upon the Beats, particularly Ginsberg. Given their affinities as poets, it seems natural to compare Whitman's relationship to food and eating with that of Ginsberg, the self-proclaimed Whitman acolyte.

Ginsberg claims Romantic poet William Blake (most famously the author of *Songs of Innocence and Experience*), who visited him in hallucinations, as a key influence, but the other strong poetic voice upon which he draws throughout his career is Whitman's. He clearly became tired of answering interviewers who asked him what his influences were, and so his throwaway reference to Whitman in one such interview needs to be taken with a grain of salt; he claims his indebtedness to Christopher Smart for the idea of using long verse lines, and simply credits Whitman with "another element of the long line" (Hamalian 1986, 299–300). But the connection is certainly deeper than that. We see it not only in the structure of Ginsberg's poems, with their repeated cadences and extended free-verse lines, but also in their celebratory nature, their epic focus on a vast sweep of humanity, and on their close attention to bodily details. Whitman's poems are omnisexual in a way that was not discussed openly at the time, while Ginsberg's (particularly some of the ones that were not published until later) are more direct in their celebration of homoeroticism. Whitman appears as a muse and character frequently in Ginsberg's poems, most famously in "A Supermarket in California," which I will discuss in further detail below. But he also makes an appearance in "Love Poem on Theme by Whitman," in which the speaker imagines himself lying down on a bed between a bride and a groom; in the late, very brief "Whitmanic Poem" (1995); and very directly in "I Love Old Whitman So" (1984), in which he rereads *Leaves of Grass* while in China and tips his poetic hat to "the old soldier, old sailor, old writer, old homosexual, old Christ poet journeyman" (Ginsberg 2006, 900).

Before looking any further at Ginsberg's work, though, we need a closer examination of how and where food appears in Whitman's poetry. At moments in Whitman, we see the speaker's desire to dissociate himself from the baseness of having to partake of food; in "Passage to India," he asks, "Have we not grovel'd/here long enough, eating and/drinking like mere/brutes?" (Whitman 2004, 437). In "Pioneers! O Pioneers!" he contrasts the "feasters" who "gluttonous feast," the "corpulent sleepers," with "ours the diet hard, and the blanket on the ground" (Whitman 2004, 261). The "Song of Prudence" mentions the "[p]utridity of gluttons or rum-drinkers" (Whitman 2004, 396). His use of food metaphors in a non-food context can be a puzzling sign of ambivalence toward the appetites. For example, in "Song of the Open Road," he says, "Still here I carry my old delicious burdens,/I carry them, men and women, I carry them with me wherever I go/I swear it is impossible for me to get rid of them,/I am fill'd with them, and I will fill them in return" (Whitman 2004, 179). To refer to burdens as "delicious" allows the sense of the contradictory (one's past, what one would now call one's "baggage," is both cumber-

some and at times something in which one indulges); just as one is satiated after a big meal but becomes hungry again eventually, it is easy to
sate oneself on the burdens of the past but also to know that as soon as
they are "digested," new ones reappear at life's table.

At other moments, Whitman uses the image of mealtime as an entry
into his romanticizing of the common people; in "I Sing the Body Electric," he describes "The group of laborers/seated at noon-time with/their
open dinner-kettles/and their wives waiting" (Whitman 2004, 128). As in
an impressionist painting, the lines seize a transitory moment: not the
moment of consumption, but the moment when food is about to be eaten.
The speaker is clearly an observer, not a participant; like the wives, he is
waiting in the wings while the "laborers" sit in expectation of that pause
in the day when they communicate vicariously with the loved one
through eating the food she has prepared, but also with the knowledge
that they are not fully at ease, for more work lies ahead. A key image
seems to be what in "Song of Myself" he calls "natural hunger," which on
one level translates into a hunger for nature and for being close to the
outer world, but it also implies a democracy of appetite and a plea not to
dismiss the appetites as immoral or unnatural. There is a powerful sensuality to his imagery in this poem of being "At the cider mill tasting the
sweets of the brown mash, sucking the juice through a straw/At apple-
peelings wanting kisses for all the red fruit I find" (Whitman 2004, 97).

Indeed, the pervasive imagery associated with eating in Whitman
connects the act of consumption, this "natural hunger," with the idea of
the great democracy of humankind. Whitman seems to argue in "Song of
Myself" that even those deemed unfit by a pious society should be able to
partake of what he imagines to be something like a giant table set with
the feast of life: "It is for the wicked just the same as the righteous, I make
appointments with all/ . . . The kept-woman, sponger, thief, are hereby
invited/The heavy-lipp'd slave is invited, the veneréalee is invited . . . "
(Whitman 2004, 81). The word "appointments" is striking because one
thinks of a well-appointed table, meaning that is set with beautiful linens
and silver and crockery, and lacks nothing in the way of food and condiments; perhaps there are also bowls of fruit and goblets of wine. The
speaker saying that he will "make appointments" implies that he is the
host of the feast, the one who issues the invitations to the table; the good
(i.e., morally upright) guests are relegated to the category of "the rest,"
while the allegedly evil or outcast ones are appointed more vividly into
the poem and into their chairs at the meal. Those whose sins are related
to other types of consuming—the kept-woman, sponger, thief, veneréalee—as well as the almost certainly hungry slave—are almost seen as
guests who are preferred over ordinary moral ones who, presumably, are
less appreciative of the appetites.

Ultimately, for Whitman, there is little separation between the act of
consumption and the emergence of the transcendent body. Again, in

"Song of the Open Road," considerations of social class are subsumed to a vision of a shared harvest: " . . . abstracting the feast yet not abstracting one particle of it/To take the best of the farmer's farm and the rich man's elegant villa/ . . . and the fruits of orchards and flowers of gardens . . . " (Whitman 2004, 187). Just as the poem itself does, the speaker feels free to appropriate—to consume—whatever is available from the best of the farmer's bounty; the "fruits" and "flowers" evoke an Edenlike milieu in which the consequences of all this taking are as yet unforeseen. The lines "abstracting the/feast yet not abstracting/one particle of it" are especially evocative of Whitman's simultaneously earthbound and transcendent view; we are asked to envision the feast, the act of eating, as something quite real—and yet, as enacted again by the poem itself, we are also asked to see it in its metaphysical state, as a sense of what it might mean if we were truly able to take in, to embody, all that is offered to us.

Consuming, in other words, becomes in Whitman an act that forges not just the link that humans have with other humans, but the link between the natural and the supernatural world. The body becomes transcendent precisely and paradoxically through the acknowledgment of its embodiment, of its hungers and appetites: "I know perfectly well my own egotism," he says in "Song of Myself": "Know my omnivorous lines and must not write any less" (Whitman 2004, 112). Finally for Whitman, to eat or to "swallow" is a means of characterizing the taking in of otherness and the change in the spiritual self that results; as he says, again in "Song of Myself," "All this I swallow, it tastes good, I like it well, it becomes mine."

While food becomes part of transcendence in Whitman, it doesn't ever leave its earthbound qualities behind in Ginsberg; indeed, his relationship with eating seems to become more and more politically charged as we follow the trajectory of his work. Eating for Ginsberg means taking in the world, as it does for Whitman, but it is also a form of anger and transgression. In an early poem, "In Society" (1947), he imagines himself at a gay cocktail party in a tiny apartment where his conversational overtures are being rebuffed; when he is offered something to eat, he says, "I ate a sandwich of pure meat; an/enormous sandwich of human flesh" which he also notices "included a dirty asshole" (Ginsberg 2006, 11). By the end of the poem, he has finally gained the attention of everyone in the room by calling a female party guest who has insulted him a "narcissistic bitch" (Ginsberg 2006, 11). Sensuality in these early works is caught up in the hunger of rejection; in "Hymn" (1949), he evokes "liturgies of milk and sweet cream sighing no longer for the strawberries of the world" (Ginsberg 2006, 44). In a manner that prefigures *Howl*, his characters in these early poems are scrambling to have enough to eat; in "Two Boys Went into a Dream Diner" (1950), the young men of the title eat five dollars (a lot) of food but have no money, yet have no idea how long it will take them "to work off what it cost" (Ginsberg 2006, 63).

Howl (1955), Ginsberg's most celebrated poem, is of course his ode to the peers of his generation. The poem is filled with references to consumption, but *what* the madmen/artists addressed and celebrated eat (in homage to Carl Solomon) in Part One of the poem is not quite literally edible: "who ate fire in paint hotels or drank turpentine in Paradise" (Ginsberg 2006, 134); "who ate the lamb stew of the imagination or digested the crab at the muddy bottom of the rivers of Bowery" (Ginsberg 2006, 136). The figures to whom he pays tribute in the poem are both literally and metaphorically hungry; the search for "jazz or sex or soup" puts all three of these things on an equal plane (Ginsberg 2006, 135). Those who inhabit this world of the artist or visionary living on the fringes of society conflate what they eat with what they create: their sustenance, probably meager in a literal sense, becomes inextricably connected to the "cooking" and "eating" of their art. What they live on now has been discarded by others as offal or is the not-yet-trendy ethnic food of the lower East Side—"who cooked rotten animals lung heart feet tail borsht and tortillas"—but while their bodies consume whatever they can get, they are "dreaming of the pure vegetable kingdom" (Ginsberg 2006, 137). The image of how these visionaries "plunged themselves under meat trucks looking for an egg" (Ginsberg 2006, 137) is highly evocative: they take huge risks, they survive on what has been rejected by others, and they follow the hope of finding the egg, the embodiment of new life, the perfect idea—however absurd the place may be in which they hope to locate it. And part I of *Howl* ends with a food image that suggests a kind of violent transubstantiation in which the works or experiences of the visionaries themselves are offered sacrificially: "with the absolute heart of the poem of life butchered out of their own bodies good to eat a thousand years" (Ginsberg 2006, 139). It is worth noting as well that food imagery drops out entirely from the remaining sections of the poem, as if its movement from the bodily experience of part I into the "Moloch" section, the apostrophe to Carl Solomon, and the final benediction in which all is "Holy" marks a movement outward and away from physical hunger into the realm of the spiritual.

According to Bill Morgan, after the famous Six Gallery performance of *Howl* in October 1955, Ginsberg read everything that he could by Whitman, and committed himself to the idea of a Whitmanlike "spontaneous method of composition" (which involved, of course, the long verse lines) as well as the Whitman-inspired use of the direct speaker/narrator (Morgan 2007, 210). To this, John Whalen-Bridge adds that the element of performance became increasingly important to him after this point (Whalen-Bridge 2016, 27). One could certainly argue that while there is a certain hubris in Ginsberg's self-positioning at this point as a young oracular voice that dares to imitate Whitman's style, his dialogue with Whitman is always a playful, comic, even self-abnegating one.

Whitman wrote on various occasions about California, calling "Song of the Redwood-Tree" a "California song" (Whitman 2004, 235), and saying in "A Promise to California," "I know very well that I and robust love belong among you, inland, and along the Western sea" (Whitman 2004, 162). And Ginsberg's most obviously known "food poem," if one may call it that, is of course "A Supermarket in California." From the beginning of this piece, which he addresses directly to Whitman ("What thoughts I have of you tonight, Walt Whitman" [Ginsberg 2006, 144]), he immediately contrasts the "neon fruit supermarket" (Ginsberg 2006, 144) of 1955 to Whitman's America. Sallie Tisdale, in *The Best Thing I Ever Tasted*, talks about the rise of the American supermarket, calling it "a playing field for a competition of equals, a stadium of attractively, almost hypnotically designed packages, containing essentially the same food and each brand promising essentially the same experience" (Tisdale 2000, 60). In Ginsberg's poem, the speaker imagines Whitman's reactions to the plentitude and to the extent to which *this* is what has become of the dream of the common feasting ground; the tone is celebratory, but with a taste of sarcastic humor: "What peaches and what penumbras! Whole families shopping at night! Aisles full of husbands! Wives in the avocadoes, babies in the tomatoes!—and you, Garcia Lorca, what were you doing down by the watermelons?" (Ginsberg 2006, 144). Whitman's natural world and Lorca's surrealism have merged into the superrealism, shades of Edward Hopper, of the America that by necessity becomes Ginsberg's own artistic inspiration. He both teases Whitman for his outsider sexuality and identifies with it, describing him as "poking among the meats in the refrigerator and eyeing the grocery boys" (Ginsberg 2006, 144). Whitman, in the speaker's imagination, is a partner in simultaneously enjoying and subverting this consumer culture: he pictures them "together in our solitary fancy tasting artichokes, possessing every frozen delicacy" (Ginsberg 2006, 144). Yet he also says that they are "followed in my imagination by the store detective" and at one point remarks feeling "absurd" (Ginsberg 2006, 144) when he pictures this supermarket adventure. By the end of the poem, he asks how the America of the 1955 supermarket compares to the visions that Whitman had, calling for guidance from his muse: "Which way does your beard point tonight?" (Ginsberg 2006, 144). At the same time that the poem professes an ambivalence about its own materials—the frozen food, the pork chops—it revels in using those same materials, those same food products, in an implicit answer to Whitman that we use what we find when we are in our "hungry fatigue and shopping for images" (Ginsberg 2006, 144). In "A Strange New Cottage in Berkeley," another California poem written around the same time as *Howl* and "A Supermarket," Ginsberg takes on a Whitmanesque voice (and yet perhaps also invokes William Carlos Williams) when he concludes the poem with the garden feeding him "its plums from the form of a small tree in the corner,/an angel thoughtful of my stomach, and my dry and lovelorn tongue" (Ginsberg 2006, 143).

The relationship with food takes a more clearly political turn in Ginsberg's poems of the 1980s and 1990s. Non-mindful consumption, for him, becomes associated with corruption; the short piece "Irritable Vegetable" from 1982 ends, "You're a jerk/You're a hypocrite who eats hot dogs" (Ginsberg 2006, 877). His 1983 "Brown Rice Quatrains" from *White Shroud* offers what we might see now as a prescient warning about the violations of integrity occurring within our food system. Whereas "Supermarket in California" at least partially celebrated consumer plenitude, "Brown Rice Quatrains" depicts a society in which what we eat is controlled by the workings of diabolical government forces: "secret police maintained ham and eggs" (Ginsberg 2006, 887). Although there is still some comedy in the deliberately histrionic and surreal phrasing of the lines, the point that we are failing to pay heed to the animal kingdom is clear: "What tragedy for multiple Chickens/Think how pigs dream butcher night!/Sheep squawked nightmare, goat/Fish sent regrets from meadow and sea" (Ginsberg 2006, 887). The pastoral has been replaced by the chemical and by the utter conflation of what we eat with the addictions bred by commercials: "Sugar dances at the movies, coffee tells you on TV/and Sodium Nitrate and Nicotine Cholesterol" (Ginsberg 2006, 887).

Like Whitman, Ginsberg provides a full palate of details; his 1984 poem "One Morning I Took a Walk in China" paints for us vividly the foods he sees as he approaches the market, with "Long green cabbages," "Leeks in a pile," and "bright orange carrots thick and rare" (Ginsberg 2006, 903). This is followed by lines describing in rather gruesome detail the meat he sees being butchered, the "half pig on a slab" and the "meat of the ox going thru a grinder, white fat red muscle & sinew together squeezed into human spaghetti" (Ginsberg 2006, 903). As he did in *Howl*, Ginsberg refuses to prettify the imagery of consumption or of how food is made; the result is that while Whitman's food imagery is never particularly graphic, Ginsberg's always reminds us of the brutality of an animal nature, of humans as animals who consume other animals.

The emphasis on consumerism and greed as portrayed through the eating of meat and animal-like behavior emerges clearly in a late (1993) poem entitled "C'mon Pigs of Western Civilization Eat More Grease," and the title says it all. The entire poem is a detailed list of decadent menu items that ooze and drip: "Buttered veal medallions in creamy saliva,/buttered beef, by glistening mountains/of french fries" (Ginsberg 2006, 1071). As the poem continues, he seems to be commanding the reader to go all-out in terms of gluttony: "order a plate of Bratwurst, fried frankfurters,/ couple billion Wimpys,' McDonald's burgers/to the moon & burp!" (Ginsberg 2006, 1071). All of this, he reveals with no small amount of sarcasm, reflects the Western world's supposed preeminence:

"Set an example for developing nations, salt/sugar, animal fat" (Ginsberg 2006, 1072). At the end of the poem, he draws a connection between "carnivorous nations" (Ginsberg 2006, 1072) and the murder going on in (at the time of the poem) countries like "Bosnia, Cypress [*sic*], Ngorno Karabach Georgia" (Ginsberg 2006, 1072). After he delivers this admonition, he closes the poem powerfully with the implication that the readers, caught up in their own gluttony, will ignore him and keep consuming those who have less power; he says, "have another coffee,/here's a cigar./ And this is a plate of black forest chocolate cake,/you deserve it" (Ginsberg 2006, 1072).

This is not to say that he ever risks taking himself too seriously, particularly in the last two decades of his writing. In "Hard Labor," we find him at Kiev, a popular East Village Ukrainian restaurant, where the Communist ideals of his early poems (like "America") take somewhat of a self-mocking turn as they become confused with the act of consumption: "The Kasha Mushrooms tastes good/as Byelorussia usta when my momma/ran away from Cossacks 1905" (Ginsberg 2006, 948). He both claims his heritage as a Jew of Eastern European descent, as well as his own political lineage as a well-known leftist, and gently pokes fun at the way he has ended up in a New York City diner. After he asks, "Did the 5 year plan work?" (Ginsberg 2006, 948)—and it's worth noting that the poem predates the supposed fall of the Iron Curtain—at the end of the poem he depicts himself as "a fairy with purple wings and white halo/translucent as an onion ring in/the transsexual fluorescent light of Kiev/Restaurant after a hard day's work" (Ginsberg 2006, 948). He makes fun of his own status as a gay man, which is both marginalized and magical, but also ultimately is like an everyday onion ring. The clever line break between "Kiev" and "Restaurant" underscores the distance between himself and his ancestors, but always with a sense of both longing for a (political?) past that is impossible to recover, and a sardonic feeling of the inevitable dissolution of political ideals in the present day.

Even though there is a clear cynicism and social critique here that takes Ginsberg's work in a different direction, this is not to suggest that he ever fully rejects Whitman's visions. The last two lines of a piece called "Big Eats" dated 8/20/91 provides a fascinating counterpart to Whitman's "All this I swallow, it tastes good, I like it well, it becomes mine" cited earlier from "Song of Myself." Ginsberg writes: "Sooner or later let go what you loved hated or shrugged off, you walk in the park/You look at the sky, sit on a pillow, count up the stars in your head, get up and eat" (Ginsberg 2006, 1011).

It's a telling moment. On the one hand, there is a surrendering of the self to the cosmos, much as Whitman might have done, with contemplation of the stars in the sky. On the other hand, there is a return to the mundane, to the bodily world. I would argue that eating here is now infused with a continuation of the celebratory, a rejoining of the spiritual with the material world: it will be an act of mindful eating that reflects the taking in of the stars in the sky. Remaining in Ginsberg, then, we find these moments of using food and eating—from a Buddhist as well as a transcendentalist point of view—to achieve a oneness with the universe. At the same time, though, I'd hasten to add in closing that his poetry of this period nevertheless carries an un-Whitman-like uneasiness with what journalist Michael Pollan later referred to as "the omnivore's dilemma." Finally, this tension between food as an everyday (required) act to be celebrated in its attention to the body, and food as the path to some kind of spiritual transcendence that goes far beyond food itself is a productive one worth keeping in mind as we move beyond Ginsberg and Whitman to the less quixotic significance of food in texts about the Holocaust.

TWO

The Politics of Gluttony in Second-Generation Holocaust Literature

Food becomes a more vital issue, obviously, when one has experienced starvation. Among writers who are the children of concentration camp survivors (also known as second-generation "survivors of survivors"), literal and figurative representations of eating too much or too little become significant markers of trauma. For the children of Holocaust survivors—now adults—who have contributed a growing body of literature to Holocaust studies, food (so obviously denied in the camps) is a vexed issue, a source of frequent confrontation. After a brief example of second-generation Holocaust poetry, I will use an historical cookbook (*In Memory's Kitchen*) to illustrate further what food meant to those incarcerated in concentration camps. Then, I will turn to two significant works about second-generation survivorship, both of which initially received controversial receptions by audiences who felt that the subject of the Holocaust was sacrosanct: Art Spiegelman's graphic memoir *Maus*, and Donald Margulies's play *The Model Apartment*. I suggest that for second-generation survivors, guilt and confusion as the result of being presented with an excess of food (and the concomitant demand that it not be wasted), in light of the parents' experience of starvation, is a common experience. As performance artist Deb Filler, whose father survived Auschwitz, remarks, "We children feel we have no voice. Because what we have experienced is in no way as significant as what our parents did. How do you beat Auschwitz? How do you beat that story?" (qtd. in Smith 1997).

Interviews with concentration camp survivors like Daniel Davidoff have frequently documented their obsession with food, both in the camps, and in their intent to consume it in abundance but without waste in the subsequent years:

Listen . . . we were like animals. We were thinking twenty-five hours a day of food. All the time food. I had a dream all the time. If I go home again, I will have a jar of cookies on my desk and I will have it any time I want it. (qtd. in Hass 1996, 98)

In Aaron Hass's important study *The Aftermath: Living with the Holocaust*, his interviewees talk often about their troubled relationships with food and eating. Hass comments, "For most survivors, the Holocaust was a thousand days of hunger, a thousand daydreams of food (a commodity worth countless gambles with one's life)." He continues by quoting two more interview subjects:

"Food, I'm different from your average person," Ida Koch told me. "I would never throw away food. I eat too much. When I was in concentration camp, my only wish was if I ever have a whole bread for myself., I would be the happiest person in the world. I ruin my health with food. I'm not going to deprive myself if I feel like something." Saul Halpern is also influenced by his previous cravings. "I'm afraid of hunger. If I buy bread, I always buy two so I shouldn't be without it." And while it has been forty-five years since Saul's stomach was empty, once again the survivor cautiously anticipates a repetition of history. (Hass 1996, 60–61)

Second-generation poet Stewart Florsheim is a helpless observer of his survivor father's eating habits: "He finishes his entire meal,/eats the ice-cream, too,/whether or not he is hungry,/if it's part of the daily special" (Florsheim 1989, 78–79). Elizabeth Rosner begins her prose poem "Disobedient Child" with the words, "No I will not eat chicken again or finish what's on my plate," and continues, "Don't tell me I know nothing about suffering just because at my age Mom was hiding from the Nazis and living on potato peels . . . ." (Rosner 1998, 35). The speaker's experiences of adolescent anguish feel impossibly diminished each time she is reminded of what her mother went through: "I won't carry your pain like it belongs to me because it's yours yours yours I have enough of my own and it's thanks to you" (Rosner 1998, 35). Even watching her mother eat becomes a painful reminder of duty, religion (the Jewish Sabbath) and past hunger: "I hate staying home with the family on Friday nights to eat chicken again and listen to Mom crack open the bones with her teeth so she can suck out the marrow" (Rosner 1998, 35). Viscerally, the speaker feels as if she is the one having the marrow sucked out of her. The very act of voicing anger about this sense of diminishment is considered inappropriate, outrageous: again, the work of art becomes a transgressive outlet. Near the end of the poem we see the fantasy of causing pain to the mother by means of food violations, even of disobeying kosher laws, mixed into a kind of imagined sexual abandon: "when someone offers me shrimp or lobster I'll say yes yes yes" (Rosner 1998, 36).

In Memory's Kitchen (1996) is a fascinating, difficult book to categorize. It consists mostly of recipes, and yet it is not a cookbook in the sense that the recipes are not really meant to be replicated. Rather, this is an oral history of sorts, a collection of recipes written by the women who were imprisoned at Terezín (Theresienstadt), the so-called model concentration camp established by the Nazis for propaganda purposes. It came to life in the form of a document that second-generation survivor Anny Stern, after twenty-five years of searching for it, received in the mail through a circuitous series of connections. Her mother, Mina Pachter, had compiled the book but had died in her seventies while still a prisoner in Theresienstadt. When Anny received it, according to Cara de Silva's introduction to the volume, it was a "fragile, hand-sewn copy book . . . its cracked and crumbling pages covered with recipes in a variety of faltering scripts" (de Silva 1996, xxv). These women had no access to the ingredients in the recipes; rather, they used conversation about the preparation of their favorite dishes as a survival strategy to give them hope and to keep their minds active. To understand this collection is to get a stronger sense of what, exactly, food meant to the inmates of the camps, and what impact this had upon their children in the next generation.

Those imprisoned at Theresienstadt included Jews whose prominent place in the arts, sciences, or business worlds meant that they were in the public eye, and so the Nazis were being careful about how their treatment was being perceived by the outside world. Although Theresienstadt was often referred to as a model camp, it's important to understand that although there were indeed many cultural events, the inhabitants (a) were there against their will, (b) were forced to pretend for visitors that things were better than they really were, and (c) were facing near-starvation conditions and poor sanitation, inadequate clothing, and overcrowded sleeping quarters, nearly as badly as in the other camps. Michael Berenbaum, director of the United States Holocaust Research Institute, puts it thus in his Foreword to the volume:

> The Nazis artfully positioned it as a model ghetto, a place that purported to demonstrate the Führer's decency to the Jews. However, in reality, it was a means of camouflaging the Reich's actual intentions in order to conceal them from an inquiring world. Behind this Potemkin village, this stage set, Theresienstadt was riddled with fear, disease, and death. This duality, along with the feverish cultural life organized by those interned there, gave the ghetto an almost surrealistic quality. (de Silva 1996, ix)

For the sake of the public eye, the Nazis allowed sanctioned arts-related events to transpire at Theresienstadt, though the prisoners needed to make sure that what they presented was not obviously subversive or overly revelatory about camp conditions, and so their performance works often had coded meanings, and painters hid their more transgressive paintings behind the walls. What is remarkable is the extent to which, by putting on plays and operas, by painting and performing music, and by writing, these prisoners were able to sustain some strength by using their imaginations to envision a future.

This was as true for the exchange of recipes as it was for more overtly art-related activities. It may sound strange that food was such a frequent topic of conversation in the camp, given the lack of it: one would think that avoiding all mention of it would help them to deal with the meagerness of their rations. There were several factors at play here, though. One was that it's important to realize that for these women in their normal (pre-camp) lives, many of whom were Czech Jews from higher social positions, cooking and eating consumed many hours of the day. As de Silva puts it, "[t]o a degree that may be unfathomable to Americans at the end of the twentieth century, cooking, both doing it and talking about it, was central to the societies from which many of the women of Terezín, and most European women of the period, came" (de Silva 1996, xxxi). Another factor was that their coping strategy involved focusing not on the horrors in front of them, but on a combination of nostalgia for the past and a hope of reemerging from the present into some kind of normalcy. And it helped to occupy the time. They took it very seriously; anecdotes from survivors mention that since the women obviously had no way to test their recipes or verify the measurements, ingredients, or cooking times, they would argue for hours about the fine details of how to prepare some dishes. This is why the book sometimes features more than one version of a recipe for a single dish, or features dishes by various names that appear to be very similar to one another. The volume's translator, Bianca Steiner Brown, who was also a prisoner at Terezín, provides a useful explanation for what it meant to be talking about food all of the time: "In order to survive, you had to have an imagination . . . You knew how it was, but you imagined it even better than it was, and that's how it was with food, also. Talking about it helped you" (de Silva 1996, xxviii). De Silva adds that we may find it difficult to understand how it could be that "people who were undernourished, even starving, not only reminisced about favorite foods but also had discussions, even arguments, about the correct way to prepare dishes they might never be able to eat again" (de Silva 1996, xxviii). Indeed, Steiner Brown says that they would often share things like cake recipes in their bunks late at night. And de Silva quotes Susan E. Cernyak-Spatz, a survivor of both Terezín and Auschwitz, as saying that this practice was so common that they even had a term for it: "We called it 'cooking with the mouth.' . . . Everybody did it. And people got very upset if they thought you made a dish the wrong way or had the wrong recipe for it" (de Silva 1996, xxix).

As mentioned earlier, it's unlikely that readers will try to duplicate these recipes at home, but that is not the point. Although the recipes comprise the longest section of the book, they are accompanied by manuscript information, notes (a glossary), and even poems and letters written by the book's original compiler. When one looks over the recipes, it's easy to see missing information or parts that were illegible (for example, the recipe for "Milk-Cream Strudel" omits instructions for the actual strudel pastry [de Silva 1996, 59], but those parts are preserved as such, even including errors in grammar or punctuation. (As de Silva points out, although the recipes are in German, it's also true that for many of the inmates who offered contributions here, German wasn't their native language [de Silva 1996, xlii].) It's also striking that many, many of the recipes are for sweets, pastries, dumplings, and other rich and filling luxury foods which it must have been a source of comfort to imagine or remember. Many of them are for traditional Jewish foods or foods with specifically Jewish labels, such as the "Cheap Real Jewish Bobe" (de Silva 1996, 19); including these would have been particularly fraught, given that the inmates were being punished for their religious beliefs. And some of the recipes are clearly designed for hard times, such as the "War Dessert," which is made from boiled potatoes (de Silva 1996, 53); it would appear that one of the subjects for discussion was how, given shortages and rationing (or more directly, the total unavailability of many foodstuffs), one could create appetizing desserts, for example. The message here was clear: even when being forced to surrender their possessions and to split apart from their loved ones, no one could take away their ability to create, even if just in their minds, the idea of making things to feast upon. Berenbaum's Foreword provides an eloquent description of the significance that sharing these recipes had for these women:

> For some, the way to deal with this hunger was to repress the past, to live only in the present, to think only of today, neither of yesterday nor of tomorrow. Not so the women who compiled this cookbook. They talked of the past; they dared to think of food, to dwell on what they were missing—pots and pans, a kitchen, home, family, guests, meals, entertainment. Therefore, this cookbook, compiled by the women in Theresienstadt, must be seen as yet another manifestation of defiance, of a spiritual revolt against the harshness of given conditions. It is a flight of the imagination back to an earlier time when food was available, when women had homes and kitchens and could provide a meal for their children. The fantasy must have been painful for the authors. Recalling recipes was an act of discipline that required them to suppress their current hunger and to think of the ordinary world before the camps—and perhaps to dare to dream of a world after the camps. (de Silva 1996, xv–xvi)

De Silva echoes this sense of the book's creation as a form of "defiance" against the idea that there was no hope and no future for survival, as well as defiance against the Nazi idea that they were subhuman and did not deserve the so-called luxury of fine cuisine. She says, "certainly the creation of such a cookbook was an act of psychological resistance, forceful testimony to the power of food to sustain us, not just physically but spiritually" (de Silva 1996, xxvi).

This is important to consider when we return to the subject of the second-generation survivors, not only the descendants of these women (including the editor of the collection) who are the heirs of these recipes, but also the readers of that volume who may or may not be second-generation survivors themselves. To read these recipes is to understand, first, what utter importance food and eating had for the inmates, not just for the purpose of everyday survival but for the purpose of being able to imagine a life beyond the camps. It helps us to recognize why, for those who survived and had children of their own, there was often an obsession with eating, with not wasting food, and with surveying their children's eating habits so closely that it often made them feel uncomfortable. But it also gives us a source of empathy, as these recipes provide such powerful testimony that their literal hunger was also a hunger for survival.

Art Spiegelman's award-winning two-volume graphic (comic book) memoir about his father, *Maus*, takes on the project of simultaneously giving us the testimonial of a survivor and the impact of having had a survivor as a parent. In an essay on the work, Michael G. Levine sees the difficulty of second-generation writers like Spiegelman as not only one of figuring out how to help their parents tell their stories, but also of "coming to terms with their own implication in their parents' experiences" (Levine 2003, 63). Anyone who has read *Maus* will recall young Artie not being permitted to leave the dinner table until he has cleaned his plate—or if he does leave, the same food will be waiting there at the next meal: "Mom would offer to cook something I liked better, but Pop just wanted to *leave* the leftover food around until I ate it. Sometimes he'd even *save* it to serve again and again until I'd eat it or starve" (Spiegelman 1986, 43). Even the opening sequence of the work involves an association of food and the horror of the past, as Artie's father, Vladek, in response to Artie being bullied on the playground as a child, says, "Friends? . . . If you lock them together in a room with no food for a week . . . THEN you could see what it is, friends!" (Spiegelman 1986, 6). As Hamida Bosmajian argues, this essentially diminishes Artie's experience because it can never be of the same magnitude as his father's: it implies "not only that friends are unreliable but also that his pains are unimportant and that he is insignificant in relation to Vladek and his story" (Bosmajian 2003, 35).

So much of Vladek's devastating narrative about his experiences hiding from the Nazis, and later in Auschwitz, returns to the idea of what one had to do to get food, from selling goods on the black market when they are in the ghetto, to feeling constant hunger when he and his wife Anja are in hiding. When he goes foraging for food and returns only with a few turnips and a bag of books, he says, "All the time we were hungry.

We just didn't have what to eat" (Spiegelman 1986, 112). At one point, everyone wants to buy a piece of his cousin Pesach's cake, since "for *years* we didn't see any cake" —but when it turns out that what he thought was flour was actually laundry soap, "we were, all of us, sick like dogs" (Spiegelman 1986, 119). When Anja becomes intolerably hungry, Vladek gives her a piece of wood to chew on, saying that "it feels a little like eating food" (Spiegelman 1986, 123). And when he is imprisoned in Po-land (just prior to when he and Anja are separate in Auschwitz) and gets a little package of food in recompense for helping a Polish prisoner to write a letter in German, he gives it to Anja and pretends he isn't hungry.

Vladek gives a detailed description of the food—or lack of it—that he and the other prisoners had when they were taken captive in the Ausch-witz concentration camp. This also helps us to understand why he is constantly having to "organize" extra food, for the inmates are being starved to death. Vladek says:

> Everybody was so hungry always, we didn't know even what we are doing. In the morning for breakfast we got only a bitter drink made from roots . . . One time a day they gave a soup from turnips. To stand near the first of the line was no good. You got only water. Near the end was better. Solid things to the bottom floated. But too far to the end it was also no good. Because many times it could be no soup anymore. And one time each day they gave us a small bread, crunchy like glass. The flour they mixed with sawdust together—we got one little brick of this what had to last the full day. Most gobbled it right away, but always I saved a half for later. And in the evening we got a spoiled cheese or jam. If we were lucky a couple times a week we got a sausage big like two of my fingers, only this much we got. If you ate how they gave you, it was just enough to die more slowly. (Spiegelman 1991, 49)

Vladek's narrative here dovetails with the ways that other survivors have described the rations in Auschwitz, and in that sense, this and many other portraits of life in the camp go beyond the personal memoir and into historical testimony from a generation from which there are now very few survivors still alive.

On an individual level, we understand increasingly as the two vol-umes of the memoir unfold that Vladek was exceptionally shrewd and forward-thinking—the way he saves half of his bread, some of which he is able to smuggle over to Anja in her camp, is only a small example— and yet, as many have pointed out, the likelihood for survival was deter-mined by sheer luck (not being in the wrong place at the wrong time), not merely by one's wits. When he is able to arrange a secret meeting with Anja, he urges her to have the same mindset; when she says that she got a job in the kitchen and brings scraps to her friends, Vladek admonishes her, "Don't worry about friends. Believe me, they don't worry about you. They just worry about getting a bigger share of your food!" (Spiegelman 1991, 56). Anja protests that she has little appetite and her friends are always hungry, but he urges her to keep up her strength. And later, when he is put into a boxcar from which very few emerge alive, he is able to stay alive by trading some of the snow to drink that he can scrape from his high perch for someone else's sugar. His narrative helps us to understand the extremities of behavior that hunger caused, such as later, in Dachau, when "if someone got soup and someone *spilled* him a drop . . . like wild animals they would fight until there was blood. You can't know what it is, to be hungry" (Spiegelman 1991, 91). The paradox is that at times, it is through appropriately aimed "friendship" behavior that Vladek is able to gain food for survival; when in Dachau he ends up in a barrack where they are given nothing to eat, he helps to bring comfort to a non-Jewish French prisoner who can't find anybody who speaks the same language by speaking English with him; in return, the French man shares his package of Red Cross provisions with him, and Vladek says that this saved his life. He even goes a step further and trades some of the chocolate for a clean shirt that he can wear only for lice inspections (prisoners with lice were turned away from the day's ration of soup), helping "the Frenchman" (which is what he calls him instead of "my friend") to do the same (Spiegelman 1991, 94). And even when he catches typhus and is too weak to eat, he trades his bread to pay for help going to the toilet.

In the present, Vladek is so badly damaged that when Francoise remarks that it's a miracle he survived, Artie's response is that "in some ways he *didn't* survive," which is entirely true (Spiegelman 1991, 90). He still compulsively saves everything he finds, like bits of string or wire or old calendars. His second wife, Maya, complains bitterly to Artie that Vladek is too cheap to give her any money for necessities like clothes. She says, "He has hundreds of thousands of dollars in the bank, and he lives like a pauper! He grabs paper towels from rest rooms so he won't have to buy napkins or tissues!" (Spiegelman 1986, 132). In *Maus II*, when Artie and his wife Francoise come to see Vladek at his bungalow in the Catskills, Vladek complains bitterly that Mala opened a container of salt when another one was only half-empty. When Francoise asks him if he wants some tea, he responds that he can reuse a tea bag from breakfast that he has drying near the sink. When his narrative to Artie distracts him and he accidentally breaks a dish, he won't let Artie throw it away, saying that he can glue it back together. When he tries to give Artie a half-eaten box of cereal and a piece of fruitcake to take home and Artie says that he doesn't want them, Vladek is insistent: "Ever since Hitler I don't like to throw out even a crumb," to which Artie responds in frustration, "Then just SAVE the damn Special K in case Hitler ever comes back!" (Spiegelman 1991, 78). Readers might particularly recall Artie's subsequent horror at watching his father attempt to return that same partially empty box of cereal to the grocery store. Artie says it's embarrassing and that he'll wait in the car; Vladek responds, "What's to be so ashamed? It's foods I can't eat. You wait then in the car while I arrange it" (Spiegelman 1991, 89). When he returns to the car, he explains with some complacency that the grocery store manager was perfectly willing to take back the cereal box after Vladek told him about the camps; Artie is beleaguered by his father's willingness to exploit his own past for the sake of economy—"We can't ever show our faces here again" (Spiegelman 1991, 90)—but we also understand that this kind of bargaining and hoarding skill is partly what kept Vladek alive in the camps in the first place. Much of the energy of the present-day portions of the memoir, then, is caught up in Artie's frustration at his father. As Nancy K. Miller suggests, "[t]he anger Vladek inspires in his son is palpable in the narrative frames in which Vladek's post-Holocaust manias are thoroughly detailed, but it also shapes Art's representation of the Holocaust testimony itself" (Miller 2003, 48). It leaves Artie in an impossible position: he feels ashamed of his father's behavior, and yet because Holocaust experience is considered sacrosanct, he has no outlet for these feelings (except of course, eventually, in the pages of this graphic memoir).

In Hass's interviews, he finds ample evidence of these kinds of struggles over food between parents and children. One second-generation survivor, Marsha, says:

> My mother's experience with deprivation has made her obsessed with food. I remember having eggs rammed down my throat and vomiting them up, and then having more shoved down again. My mother is always thinking about, talking about, cooking, freezing, or packaging food. As a result, I was the closest thing to anorexic as a child without being one. I didn't really start eating until I went away to college. (qtd. in Hass 1990, 61)

Marsha's real-life drama is not too far away from the works of playwrights like Georg Tabori and Donald Margulies, both of whom are examples of artists who stage this conflict over food; for the rest of this discussion, I want to consider Margulies's controversial second-generation Holocaust play *The Model Apartment*. Although Margulies brings up Jewishness as a theme in other works—such as *The Loman Family Picnic*, where the father and son fight over the son's bar mitzvah money—his most direct approach to food and other issues in a post-Holocaust context is in *The Model Apartment*.

I saw *The Model Apartment* in production at Second Stage in New York City in 1995. One thing I recall quite vividly is being seated next to a woman in the audience who had survived the Holocaust herself, gold bracelets not quite covering her tattoo, and who was very disturbed by the play's less-than-reverent approach to the issue of the wounds that survivors unintentionally inflict upon their offspring. Robert Skloot emphasizes the power of post-Holocaust drama to affect its audience by drawing upon techniques that are "without sentimentality" (Skloot 1988, xvi). And as Vivian Patraka puts it, Margulies's play "raises the question of how realism itself can be reconfigured to disrupt the very narrative of expectations that come from the form, in this case by making us persistently uncomfortable about how we conceive of survivors" (Patraka 1999, 10).

At the beginning of the play, Max and Lola, both concentration camp survivors, have come down to Florida and are put up for the night in what they think will be a luxury condominium, but is what turns out to be a "model apartment," complete with fake TV set. Margulies uses this image to create the sense that the dreamed-for retirement home is merely a construction, a cardboard dream; his opening stage directions state, "Candles, ashtrays, and bric-a-brac are glued to surfaces. Objects function solely as decoration; the television and appliances are state-of-the-art but hollow" (Margulies 1995, 142). As it turns out, no refuge is possible for Max and Lola—not only because of the shared horrors of their past, but also because they are running away from their nightmarish daughter, Debby, as they feel both persecuted by her and guilty about feeling menaced by their own child.

Debby, of course, shows up—there is no escape—with her learning-disabled boyfriend, Neil, in tow. She is both a caricature and a very real figure: "grossly obese and unkempt," she is described as "like a blimp, the Hindenburg, slowly floating, winding through the apartment" (Margulies 1995, 153). Possibly insane, she rants and raves to her parents, conflating past and present, turning their Holocaust stories (which she has been forced to ingest all her life) into attacks that are horribly tasteless and devastatingly funny. As she obsessively consumes American junk food, Debby says she feels that she is being stuffed with stories of her parents' past. While "eat[ing] out of the cereal box and guzzl[ing] milk," she tells her mother:

> The last time I visited the concentration camp, they turned it into a bungalow colony. They put chintzy drapes on the barbed wire. Raisin cookies were in the ovens. The food, Mommy! Such portions! I was stuffed! None of that stale bread and soup shit. All the salad bar you can eat! Shrimp! Like at Beefsteak Charlie's. (Margulies 1995, 165)

As in Rosner's poem, the evocation of shrimp at the end of this speech, which is distinctly non-kosher, would—one might guess—send Lola over the edge. But Lola does not react with much shock; it is clear that she has been listening to this kind of talk from her daughter for years. Debby's diatribes suggest not simply an idiosyncratic conflation of the Holocaust with contemporary junk culture (and one might remember the recent real-life controversy over the installation of a McDonald's near Dachau), but also the extent to which the "marketing" of the Holocaust *has* indeed become part of current consumerist obsessions. Debby is a grotesque caricature, but her character is also a symbol of how this era in world history risks becoming yet another commodity.

The play is complicated further by Debby's inability to fill the void created in her mother's and father's lives by the loss of their first daughter (also named Deborah), who did not survive the war. In his research on the children of survivors, indeed, Hass writes, "Those made to feel guilty invariably grow to resent that onerous burden. Themes of anger and the mishandling of that emotion have been commonly observed among [these subjects]" (Hass 1996, 28). Indeed, Artie in Spiegelman's *Maus* talks about being haunted by the photograph of his brother Richieu, who died in the Holocaust, as an image of a child frozen in time whose perfection he himself could never hope to attain. And in *The Model Apartment*, Debby confronts her father in a key moment:

> What do you want me to do, Daddy? Rip off my rolls? Tear off my skin? . . . Starve myself to death? Would that make you happy? Huh? How could I possibly be as pretty as Deborah? Skin and bones. Stick my finger down my throat. Vomit rots your teeth. Mengele was my dentist. He was Mister Wizard. He put my teeth in Coca-Cola. They burned like acid. Mengele taught you brain surgery. (Margulies 1995, 189)

Hass finds in his study that "[a] survivor's memory of a first spouse and perhaps child who were killed often overshadowed the new family indefinitely" (Hass 1996, 12). Flashbacks or ghostly haunting of a rail-thin Deborah appear frequently to Max, the father, pleading with him in Yiddish; productions of *The Model Apartment* often cast the same actress to play both Deborahs, implying that they are problematic doubles whose fate took opposite directions, and yet both of whom are outcasts or no longer part of the everyday world.

By the end of the play, Debby is taken away by ambulance, "tied up and gagged" (Margulies 1995, 191). Interestingly, the survivorship Max speaks of here has transmuted into one of Debby's indefatigability: "You don't give up. You come after us no matter what. You're amazing! We don't sleep at night, worried what you might do" (Margulies 1995, 191). Debby has taken the place of the Nazi persecutors in her parents' nightmares at the same time that she herself is a "survivor" of her own parents' past. Max and Lola are divided over the idea of how much ultimate loyalty they now owe her daughter; Lola refuses to turn her back on Debby, saying, "I can't deny her, Max. She exists" (Margulies 1995, 193). In this sense, the attempt to deny the existence of the irreverent daughter is made into a sort of Holocaust denial, even as Max himself insists upon denying the *present* and slipping back into his memories of the past.

The play concludes with Max conjuring up the image of Deborah (who actually died in infancy) in the afterlife; her monologue's final depictions of eating and hunger resonate painfully with the lingering impression of Debby, whose real-life hunger for a genuine self cannot be dissipated:

> There is so much food! The kitchen is noisy with women. The dining room is cloudy with smoke and opinions . . . I miss you all the time. The men are always arguing. And a feast is always awaiting us in the kitchen. And I'm always hungry, always hungry . . . And I can't keep my eyes open, I've sipped too much wine, and I don't want to go to sleep hungry, but my eyes are closing, they're closing, and I don't want to fall asleep and miss the feast, I don't want to miss the feast . . . (Margulies 1995, 195)

For second-generation Holocaust writers like Rosner, Spiegelman, and Margulies, gluttony is never too far from its opposite, from starvation that is remembered or actual, literal or figurative. Ultimately, in associating these images with reminders of more politicized forms of commodification, these authors invite us to consider the even fatter question of how images of the overfilled, overstuffed, and overdetermined (and their opposites) connect to the risk of the Holocaust itself becoming consumable, becoming a consumer spectacle. And as we will see in the following chapter, we "inherit" (and may choose to accept or reject) recipes from the past that we revise into the future.

THREE

Chukla Bukla

Cooking, Bengali-Indian-Anglo American
Writers, and the Merging of Cultures

Hunger and the concomitant desire to be fed, as discussed in the previous chapter, is at the heart of familial experience. This chapter looks at three emblematic Indian/Bengali texts—Anita Desai's novel *Fasting, Feasting*, the stories in Jhumpa Lahiri's *Unaccustomed Earth*, and Shelby Silas's play *Calcutta Kosher*—to show how food, hunger, and cooking become ways of wrestling with questions about postcolonialism, religion, family, and identity. I am interested in how experiences of food in these works embody larger questions about multicultural identities, social class standing, maternal relationships, and religious practices and affiliations. In all three of these works, the characters' intertwined literal and metaphorical hungers become part of their struggle to define their culture and gender positions on their own terms, even amidst their ambivalence about maintaining the traditions of an older generation.

These hungers and these struggles are central to Indian/Bengali nonfiction as well as fiction. Lahiri has also written about the power of her mother's cooking in real life, and several recent food memoirs—such as Shoba Narayan's *Monsoon Diary* and Padma Lakshmi's *Love, Loss, and What We Ate*—attest to the significance of learning to prepare the dishes of one's heritage, though the act of doing so is complicated by assumptions related to gender expectations. Lakshmi's memoir, for instance, speaks with both poignancy and some implied cultural distance about the way her grandparents' generation saw cooking and its relation to hierarchies and marriageability:

Indeed, food and femininity were intertwined for me from very early on. Cooking was the domain not of girls, but of women. You weren't actually allowed to cook until you mastered the basics of preparing the vegetables and dry-roasting and grinding the spices. You only assisted by preparing these *mise en places* for the older women until you graduated and were finally allowed to stand at the stove for more than boiling tea. Just as the French kitchens had their hierarchy of *sous-chefs* and *commis*, my grandmother's kitchen also had its own codes. The secrets of the kitchen were revealed to you in stages, on a need-to-know basis, just like the secrets of womanhood. You started wearing bras; you started handling the pressure cooker for lentils. You went from wearing skirts and half saris to wearing full saris, and at about the same time you got to make the rice batter crepes called *dosas* for everyone's tiffin. You did not get told the secret ratio of spices for the house-made *sambar* curry powder until you came of marriageable age. And to truly have a womanly figure, you had to eat, to be voluptuously full of food. (Lakshmi 2016, 45)

As with Lakshmi, the characters in these works by Desai, Lahiri, and Silas face gender-related pressures that are at times overwhelming. More often than not, the conflicts over gender roles play themselves out in dramas related to the acts of cooking and eating—and as we see in the first of these works, Desai's *Fasting, Feasting*, the gendered expectations for characters' food behavior is fraught for men as well as for women.

Desai's *Fasting, Feasting*, a finalist for the Booker Prize, was first published in 1999. The *Guardian Weekly* called Desai "Jane Austen-ish in her ruthlessness and pity" (front matter), and the comparison is rather apt. Desai has Austen's comic flair in her ability to mock her characters gently at the same time that we feel for their ineptitude or their societal struggles. The novel is divided into two distinct but related sections. In the first part, which is set in India, the focus is on Uma, the rather awkward daughter whose efforts to assert an identity are overshadowed by her dominating parents and their favoritism toward her brother Arun. In the second part of the novel, the focus shifts to Arun in Massachusetts as a college student who feels desperately out of place and who tries to make sense of the Pattons, a dysfunctional American family with whom he is boarding for the summer. This is very much a novel about social caste and class, about the conflicting gender expectations for Indian men and women, and about the funny and brutal experience of being a teenager. Underlying all of this, though, is—as the title of the novel itself suggests—a preoccupation with the polarities of fasting and feasting, of eating and not eating, and what these mean both culturally (for Indian and American characters) and individually (for our protagonists and the characters who surround them).

Several scholars have noticed the multiple meanings of the title. Ludmila Volná points out that "'fasting' and 'feasting' can stand for the two parts of the novel respectively [India and America]," but also that the "'fasting' and the 'feasting' of the individual characters is relative and multiple at the same time" (Volná 2005, 43). Angelia Poon says that the book "underscores the dialectical relationship between fasting and feasting or the entangled politics of gender and cultural inequality, and shows at times how parasitically or symbiotically subjects are placed in relation to each other" (Poon 2008, 36). Francine Prose says that the novel "makes us understand how much of our lives is encoded in — and determined by — tiny, repetitive, deceptively trivial decisions about what we will and won't eat. These minute quotidian expressions of conflict and concord, preference and identity, are . . . nearly invisible but all-important in their effect on our relations with one another, on our sense of self, on our very survival" (Prose 2000, 10).

In the first part of the novel, Uma's parents, the collective entity known as MamaPapa, spend much of their time talking about food and planning orders to give the cook. Mama tells Uma about a childhood in which special treats like nuts and sweets were reserved for boys, except when her mother or aunts would "slip us something on the sly" (Desai 2000, 6). We see immediately a world in which there are clear gender roles and clear taboos. Her parents debate one another about what to tell the cook to prepare for dinner each night, but the outcome is always the same: "if Mama had suggested plain rice and mutton curry to begin with," then that is what they would have, "no matter what fancies had been entertained along the way: pilaos, kebabs, koftas . . . " (Desai 2000, 14). We see Mama's ritual peeling of an orange for Papa, as each segment of it is "peeled and freed of pips and threads till only the perfect globules of juice are left" (Desai 2000, 23), and afterwards, Papa is the only family member who has a napkin and finger bowl: "they are emblems of his status" (Desai 2000, 24). Volná reads this passage as emblematic of the patriarchal hierarchies in the novel: "Only father is feasting on power as represented by the orange, neither the mother nor Uma have any access to the orange" (Volná 2005, 44).

Male privilege is also given to Arun as a baby, as both parents monitor every bite he consumes as an infant. They develop a sort of panic over his rejection of most foods until they have to learn to accept that he is a vegetarian, a fact that bewilders Papa, who does not understand Arun's "completely baffling desire to return to the ways of his forefathers" (Desai 2000, 33). Celebrated writer J.M. Coetzee, in his piece about Desai's novel for the *New York Review of Books*, argues that Arun's vegetarianism (and his later finding of all kinds of flesh as repulsive) is "because in his being he is an ascetic, just as in her being his sister Uma is a religious devotee" (Coetzee 2000, 34). At one point while they are children, Uma bonds with Arun by sneaking him a snack of unripe guava, a food that the sickly son is forbidden by MamaPapa to consume. Arun's struggles over food become central to his experiences in America in the second half of the novel, and indeed, one of the only things he expresses in his letters home at the end of this first half is his repeated complaint that the "food is not very good" (Desai 2000, 123). Indeed, as Poon suggests, "Arun's rebelliousness is encoded in his vegetarianism, which stands in the novel as a form of passive self-assertion against the meat-eating version of hypermasculinity extolled by his father and the male members of the Patton family in the United States" (Poon 2008, 36). Indeed, Poon takes this argument a step further by arguing that since Uma is forced to take care of Arun—and at one point, as an infant, he bites her finger when she is feeding him—she is "the one on whom Arun is made to 'feast'" (Poon 2008, 39).

Uma, who is awkward and ungainly and who is expected to wait obediently upon MamaPapa at every turn, longs "hungrily" (Desai 2000, 40) for some kind of transcendence, only to be disappointed and re-pressed again and again. Whether she is joining her "aunt" (actually a distant relative) Mira-Masi in her religious rituals, shocking her parents by wanting to go to dinner at a restaurant with her cousin Ramu, or eyeing her treasured collection of Christmas cards, Uma only has room to rebel in the smallest of ways. The other young women in her extended family are, like Uma, bound by prescribed gender roles. Even her beauti-ful cousin Anamika, who has won a scholarship to Oxford, is forced into an abusive marriage where, as daughter-in-law, she ranks so low that she "spent her entire time in the kitchen" (Desai 2000, 70) cooking for her in-laws and only being allowed to eat after the men and children have had their food. While Anamika's story ends in tragedy, Uma's sister Aruna marries into a wealthier family and is given a measure of independence. Yet she is ashamed of her own relatives when she brings her in-laws for a visit and is horrified, for example, that the cook has made a salad without any dressing. Uma actually pities Aruna for having such perfectionist expectations that she can be "vexed to the point of tears because the cook's pudding had sunk and spread instead of remaining upright and solid" (Desai 2000, 109).

Even Uma becomes a victim of the gendered role of cook/housewife that is expected of her; when her parents finally find her a suitor, she is instructed to pretend that she made the samosas herself. She, too, is forced to cook for her cruel in-laws and is only rescued when it is discov-ered that her new husband was deceiving MamaPapa and already had a wife and four children. Uma returns home in shame to live with her parents again, with the understanding that she is no longer marriage material. When Uma is invited to a coffee party by her Christian friend Mrs. O'Henry, she is so grateful for the experience that she fails to under-stand the latter's thinly veiled contempt for native Indian cuisine, as Mrs. O'Henry says that she would never order her snacks from the local baker:

I order my peanut butter from Landour and the cookies are baked according to a recipe in the Landour cook book. The ladies in our mission wrote it especially for Indian conditions, you know, which are different from those at home. But they have lived in this country for a long time and they know what ingredients are available and how Indian ovens work. They've taught a local grocer to make peanut butter, and pickle relish, and blackberry jam, and other things for folks like us. It sure helps. (Desai 2000, 115)

At the end of part one of the novel, Dr. Dutt, a distinguished older unmarried woman, asks MamaPapa for permission to hire Uma as the housekeeper at her Institute, an idea which thrills Uma beyond words, but of course MamaPapa shut down the proposal instantly, and Uma is consigned once again to a life in which her longings for some kind of escape are tamped down. We then learn that her cousin Anamika has suffered an even crueler fate, having been burned to death by her husband and mother-in-law. In a final small gesture of reconciliation with Mama, while they are on the funeral boat, Uma sees Mama's tears and uses an offer of food to comfort her by saying, "I told cook to make puri-alu for breakfast" (Desai 2000, 155). In response, "Mama gives a sob and tightens her hold on Uma's hand as though she too finds the puri-alu comforting; it is a bond" (Desai 2000, 156).

The second part of the novel focuses on Arun during one summer while he is in college in the United States, a place where he feels deeply unsettled and alone. Since he does not want to live with the other Indian students, he accepts an offer to board for the summer with a suburban family, the Pattons. Much of the attention in the narrative that follows goes to Mrs. Patton, a frustrated and unhappy mother who tries to bond with Arun through grocery shopping and food (she claims that she, too, will become a vegetarian) but whose advances (which are for the most part not overtly sexual, but it is implied that she has feelings for him) make him increasingly uncomfortable. There is an odd mirroring between Arun's own family and the Pattons; for example, when Mrs. Patton tells Arun to wash his hands because "Daddy's got dinner waiting," Arun senses that her "murmur is as an order might be from another, so urgent it is, and eloquent" (Desai 2000, 163). Just as we saw Papa's discomfort with Arun's vegetarianism in part one, Mr. Patton—who is barbecuing steaks on the grill—remarks that it is "not natural" (166). Yet Arun also "wince[s]" at Mrs. Patton's overenthusiastic defense of his choice: "[s]he does not seem to have his mother's well-developed instincts for survival through evasion" (Desai 2000, 167). As Prose puts it, the Pattons "use their dietary preferences as a tool with which to form allegiances and exert power—and as a weapon with which to cause pain, to struggle for self-determination" (Prose 2000, 11). Coetzee sees the novel's struggles between vegetarians and meat-eaters as emblematic of the struggle for India's place within the developing world:

The conflict between Arun and his father is thus more than a simple family quarrel. The two stand for opposed views on what price the Hindu—and the Indian—should be prepared to pay for a place in the modern world. In his confused and utterly unheroic refusal of the beef that Mr. Patton slaps down on his plate, and more generally, in his failure to find in the New World feast the kind of food that will nourish him. Arun thus not only preserves a minimal personal integrity but stands for resistance at a precultural level, the level of the body itself: this "underdeveloped" Indian body is not and will not become an American body. (Coetzee 2000, 34)

Mrs. Patton insists that Arun accompany her on her frequent journeys to the grocery store, where he is fascinated and appalled by the various manifestations of American consumerism. At the store, Mrs. Patton is in her element, with none of the "tentativeness and timidity" (Desai 2000, 183) that she exhibits at home. It bewilders Arun to see Mrs. Patton purchase such an abundant number of groceries and to feel satisfied simply at the idea of having all of them available in the refrigerator. Since he does not know how to tell her that the kinds of foods she buys so happily—salad fixings, cereal—do not agree with his digestion, he longs for the first time for meals of the type that he was served back home in India— hence his complaints, mentioned earlier, in his letters home. Desai uses Arun's sensations of disenfranchisement to make a larger statement about the culture gap here, and about postmodern simulacra as embodied through the facsimiles of cooking and meals. In the process, Arun develops a far more complicated sense of what "home" means. Rather than escaping home, "he had stumbled into what was like a plastic representation of what he had known at home; not the real thing—which was plain, unbeautiful, misshapen, fraught and compromised—but the unreal thing—clean, bright, gleaming, without taste, savour or nourishment" (Desai 2000, 185). When Mrs. Patton suggests that Arun cook Indian food for both of them, he doesn't know how to tell her that he has no idea how, for the social class roles at home have dictated that he has never had to prepare his own meals, and that even his mother has a servant do the cooking. Yet, again, he is reminded of his own mother when he sees Mrs. Patton's facial expressions:

> She smiles a bright plastic copy of a mother-smile that Arun remembers from another world and another time, the smile that is tight at the corners with pressure . . . Mrs. Patton's smile contains no hint of pressure, it is no more than a mock-up. Gently, it flashes a message as if on a flickering screen: "Eat. Enjoy." Helplessly, he does. (Desai 2000, 194)

As the summer goes on, Arun notices that Mrs. Patton is wearing bright lipstick, lying outside in the sun in minimal clothing, and exhibiting other behaviors that make him feel very ill at ease, culminating in a grocery store trip where the cashier remarks that Mrs. Patton must be pregnant because she has a certain glow about her. All of this comes to an abrupt end, though, when Mrs. Patton finally notices something that Arun has been acutely aware of all summer: that her teenage daughter, Melanie, is suffering from bulimia. Through the character of Melanie, Desai complicates the "fasting, feasting" imagery of the title and also sets up another mirroring, this time between Melanie and Arun's sister Uma.

Although Arun never directly identifies Melanie as bulimic, the reader understands this from the very first moment that he encounters her in the bathroom, kneeling at the toilet bowl. She gorges herself on candy, telling Arun, "I'm so hungry I've got to eat this shitty candy" (Desai 2000, 195) and then engaging in ritual purging; her mother is oblivious to this problem, though when Arun says something about it to her brother Rod, he responds contemptuously, "Wants to turn herself into a slim chick. Ha!" (Desai 2000, 204). As Poon points out, bulimia inherently involves both fasting and feasting; she says that it is through Melanie's disorder that we find the "ultimate embodiment" of the "idea of emptiness in feasting" (Poon 2008, 45). When Mrs. Patton tries to get Melanie to eat scrambled eggs, we see how deeply unhappy the girl is, as she says to her mother, "Everything you cook is—poison!" (Desai 2000, 207). In a moment bordering on recognition or empathy, Arun—watching Melanie's face as she binges on ice cream—realizes where he has seen an expression like hers before:

> a resemblance to the contorted face of an enraged sister who, failing to express her outrage against neglect, against misunderstanding, against inattention to her unique and singular being and its hungers, merely spits and froths in ineffectual protest. How strange to encounter it here, Arun thinks where so much is given, where there is both license and plenty.
>   But what is plenty? What is not? Can one tell the difference? (Desai 2000, 214)

As Poon says, "Uma's spiritual, intellectual and emotional starvation finds its physical counterpart in the inexpressible hunger underlying Melanie's eating disorder" (Poon 2008, 46).

The culmination of Melanie's secret purging episodes comes when she, Mrs. Patton, and Arun visit a local swimming hole, and when Arun goes off by himself, he runs into Melanie, who is lying on the ground, very ill, covered with her vomit. Just before Mrs. Patton arrives and realizes what has been going on with her daughter, Arun tentatively puts his hand on her shoulder and asks if she needs help. As he does so, he again experiences a moment of recognition as he realizes that despite her privileges, she is really suffering: "This is no plastic mock-up, no cartoon representation such as he has been seeing all summer; this is a real pain and a real hunger. But what hunger does a person so sated feel?" (Desai 2000, 224). Guarded though Arun has been—and despite the real culture shock he has experienced—it is through his initial identification of Melanie's pain with that of his sister Uma that he approaches something like compassion. Difficult as it is for him to acknowledge that a (literally) gut-wrenching level of emotional turmoil might be possible for a privileged American teenage girl to undergo, in this moment he—and the reader as well—is forced to look beyond boundaries of gender, class, and cultural location and to understand "hunger" in a more abstract way.

At the end of the novel, as Arun prepares to return to the dorm (where he has decided to live with the other Indian students after all), we learn that Melanie has been placed in an institution for girls with eating disorders and is reportedly doing fairly well: or at least the authorities there describe her as "compliant and obedient" (Desai 2000, 227), though we never learn more of her real experiences there. As for Arun, he approaches Mrs. Patton—who has retreated into a depressed state and is reportedly planning to sign up for new-age courses in alternative medicine, astrology, and yoga, despite her husband's disapproval—and hands her tea and a shawl that his family sent him from India. As the reviewer for *Publishers Weekly* puts it, "his final act in the novel suggests both how far he has come and how much he has lost" (*"Fasting Feast"* [review] 1999). And Volná says that he "has all he needs and he has no space for the additional weight of the patriarchal baggage" (Volná 2005, 49). On the one hand, it is an unplanned gift—the items were meant to be for Arun himself—but on the other hand, there is a moment of beauty in his gesture and in Mrs. Patton's appreciation of it. She inhales the shawl's scent, which is "muddy, grassy, smoky, ashen" as her "face spreads into a flush of wonder" (Desai 2000, 228). Throughout the novel, Mrs. Patton's attempts to understand Arun's culture through his food preferences have been awkward, misguided, appropriative. For a fleeting moment at the end here, though, through the senses of smell and touch, she is able to accept his gift on its own terms—and Arun is able to give something of himself without resentment and without relinquishing his own freedom. That may be, Desai implies, the most one can ask.

Jhumpa Lahiri won the Pulitzer Prize in fiction in 1999 for her first short story collection, *Interpreter of Maladies*, and her novel *The Namesake* (2003) was made into a film in 2007. As Laura Fine points out, though Lahiri's work "isn't conventionally diasporic, the web of familial and cultural identities from which her characters unsuccessfully struggle to escape suggests that her work shares some important concerns of postcolonial literature" (Fine 2011, 212). Lahiri was born in London and grew up in Kingston, Rhode Island, but her family often visited relatives in Calcutta. When she was growing up, the procuring of ingredients for the meals her mother cooked, and the act of cooking itself, was laden with importance. Lahiri writes lovingly of the "Food Suitcase" that her parents would use to bring back spices and delicacies from Calcutta that they couldn't find in the United States in the 1970s: "Trips to Calcutta let my parents again eat the food of their childhood, the food they had been deprived of as adults" (Lahiri 2000, 184). In an essay called "The Long Way Home" that Lahiri wrote for the *New Yorker*, she recalls her mother's obsession with Indian cooking but also her refusal to share techniques with her daughter: "[C]ooking was her jurisdiction. It was also her secret. My mother owned no cookbooks, just as she owned no measuring cups or spoons" (Lahiri 2004). When Lahiri herself began to attempt to cook Indian food while she was a graduate student, "I did not ask my mother for instructions nor did she offer any" (Lahiri 2004)—instead, she turned to a Madhur Jaffrey cookbook. It was only in later years that Lahiri's mother began to let her daughter cook for extended family and friends, and only slowly did she begin to offer any advice, such as the suggestion to add a little bit of sugar to a curry.

Lahiri's fiction draws meaningfully and constantly upon images of food to illustrate issues of home, loneliness, longing, and the conflicts that her bicultural characters face. I will focus here on several of the stories in her 2009 collection *Unaccustomed Earth*. Part One of this collection features five short stories, and Part Two, "Hema and Kaushik," is a novella in the form of three linked short stories. All of the pieces in *Unaccustomed Earth* revolve around themes of family conflict, loneliness, and absent or missing characters, and in all of them, the characters, most of whom are first or second-generation immigrants from Bangladesh or India—associate food not only with nostalgia for the homeland, but also with an attempt to forge a new or emerging cultural identity. In the discussion that follows, I will focus on two of the stories in Part One, "Unaccustomed Earth" and "Hell-Heaven," and on the "Hema and Kaushik" linked stories in Part Two.

In the title story, Ruma—who is married to a white American and has a young son—is flooded with memories of her late mother when her father—who has been traveling with a secret girlfriend—comes for a visit. An early passage, in which Ruma thinks about her father's passion for gardening, is emblematic of their family dynamic. We are told that the mother often had to keep dinner waiting while the father worked in his garden, but that she would never dream of going ahead and eating without him, as she had always been trained to serve her husband before herself. In turn, the vegetables that the father grows are ones that the mother used in cooking their native dishes: special types of spinach, bitter melon, chili peppers. Their bond and struggle as described via the image of the garden reflects their immigrant status: "Oblivious to her mother's needs in other ways, he had toiled in unfriendly soil, coaxing such things from the ground" (Lahiri 2009, 16).

The brilliance of this story lies in its alternation between third-person limited narration from Ruma's and her father's points of view; as a result, we learn the secrets they are keeping from one another. The father recalls that he met Mrs. Bagchi (the woman he has been seeing) when they were on a tour together in Italy and bonded over their lack of interest in the huge lunches that the rest of the group was eating: upon being told that the lunches were optional, the two of them began to spend more time together. Yet all he tells Ruma, to answer her question about what he ate in Italy, was that he mostly ate pizza.

We realize with the shift in narrative voice that Ruma feels tremendous pressure to cook the types of Bengali dishes for her father that her mother used to make; she has spent several days prior to his visit trying to prepare the foods that she thinks he will expect. When she cooks for her husband, she can take shortcuts because he won't know the difference, but her mother "had never cut corners" (Lahiri 2009, 22) even though the only times her father showed his appreciation for her labor was in comparison to the inferior dishes they sometimes consumed as guests in other households. Now that her father is visiting, she eats, like him, with her fingers. What really strikes her, though, is that even though she knows her cooking is subpar compared to her late mother's—"the vegetables sliced too thickly, the rice overdone" (Lahiri 2009, 22)—her father keeps telling her how delicious it is.

The generational and cultural divide becomes even more apparent as Ruma's young son Akash expresses his dislike for the food that she has prepared. He eats little else but boxed macaroni and cheese, as since her mother's death she has given up on the effort to get him to like traditional Bengali cuisine. Again, the way that Ruma thinks about food represents her larger fears about the difficulty of raising her child: "he was turning into the sort of American child she was always careful not to be . . . imperious, afraid of eating things" (Lahiri 2009, 23). She deeply feels the loss of her mother as she remembers how her mother came to love Ruma's American husband and would make him the sweets called *mishti*, which Ruma herself never learned how to prepare.

The turning point of the story comes as Ruma's father begins to bond with Akash, even teaching him to count in Bengali, and the two of them spend hours together in the garden. She is surprised to see her father washing the dishes, fetching treats for Akash from a local bakery, and reading to him at night before bed. Again, though, it is mostly through food that we see the father and daughter learning to accept one another in new ways. Fatigued by her current pregnancy, she realizes that not only is her father helping with the dishes and with taking care of Akash, but at dinnertime he appreciated the American food that she began cooking again. When the father prepares to return to his own home, he accidentally leaves behind a postcard that he wrote to Mrs. Bagchi in Bengali that he had planned to mail without Ruma seeing. She finds the postcard and realizes how little she really knows about his current life, yet even as she is filled with longing for her mother and is dumbstruck by the possibility that her father has a girlfriend, the story ends with her putting the postcard into the mail for him. While the gesture of mailing the postcard represents the act of healing and the effort at cross-generational understanding, that act became possible through the ways in which moments of transformation (the father doing dishes and planting a garden for Ruma; Ruma realizing she doesn't have to cook elaborate Indian meals for her father) were created through food.

"Hell-Heaven" is a story narrated from the point of view of Usha, a woman who remembers how her mother fell in love with Pranab, a young Indian man who has been spending time with their family. Their friendship begins through food, when she finds out he has not had a "proper Bengali meal" in months (Lahiri 2009, 61) and ends up taking many of his meals with them. Pranab is from a rich family in Calcutta and has come to the United States for engineering classes at MIT; when he comes over, he eats "ravenously" (Lahiri 2009, 63), whereas the narrator's father, we're told, "disliked excess in anything" and "did not eat with the reckless appetite of Pranab" (Lahiri 2009, 65). While the father keeps to himself, Pranab—who knows the mother's home town—engages her in conversation and seems genuinely interested in what she has to say; the narrator says that she now realizes that her mother must have fallen in love with him.

When Pranab begins dating Deborah, a white woman, and brings her to dinner, the mother shows her jealousy by complaining about having to make the food less spicy. Pranab and Deborah show their affection through food—"Sometimes they ended up feeding each other, allowing their fingers to linger in each other's mouth"—which embarrasses and infuriates the mother. Eventually, the two marry, and again, we see tension as portrayed through food when the family is given fish (since they are not beef-eaters) and the father eats it awkwardly with a knife and fork (he is used to eating with his hands) while the mother declares it "inedible" (Lahiri 2009, 74). As Usha grows into adolescence, the family attends a Thanksgiving meal (even though her parents don't usually celebrate the holiday) hosted by Pranab and Deborah: again, it is through the lens of a food-related ritual celebration that we understand the characters' emotional state. Usha remarks that when they arrive, the meal is still being prepared, with dirty bowls and chaos everywhere—"something my mother always frowned upon" (Lahiri 2009, 77). When the hosts bring out the turkeys, Usha says that even though she found the food tempting, she knows that her mother would denigrate it later. Pranab compounds the mother's discomfort by saluting her in a toast, saying that the first meal he had in their household was like Thanksgiving to him. Michael Wutz suggests that in this and other stories, Lahiri "dispels Thanksgiving as the American founding myth of cross-cultural acceptance, and what should, in theory, be a meaningful dialogue among resident nations and new arrivals over a shared meal recognizing the bounty of the earth, becomes a hollow ritual leading to estrangement and distance" (Wutz 2015, 254).

Changes happen as the years pass, and eventually, Pranab divorces Deborah when he becomes involved with a married Bengali woman, and the mother seems to develop a warmer relationship with her husband (Usha's father) in their later years. The story ends with a devastating twist, though, as Usha recounts an event that her mother tells her about shortly after Usha herself has experienced a bad breakup (Lahiri 2009, 83). We learn that a few weeks after Pranab's and Deborah's wedding, the mother goes into the backyard and pours lighter fluid on her sari, planning to self-immolate: she is saved in the nick of time by a neighbor who engages her in conversation about admiring the sunset. She goes back inside, and Usha says that when she and her father arrived home a few hours later, "she was in the kitchen boiling rice for our dinner, as if it were any other day" (Lahiri 2009, 83). The revelation is a powerful one. The incident confirms the enormity of the mother's hopelessness and frustration, yet it returns to the realm of the kitchen and the ritual of meal preparation. It conveys her love for her daughter, yet the story, when shared, is more disturbing than comforting. Food is the site of transcendence but also of secret longings and secret grief.

"Hema and Kaushik," the three linked stories, again connect food imagery with nostalgia and desire. In the first story, which focuses on Hema as a girl and her initial impressions of Kaushik, the son of her parents' friends, we immediately see Hema's mother cooking eggplant and dal in preparation for the arrival of Kaushik's family to their home in the United States (Lahiri 2009, 231). As this narrative develops, we see Hema's fascination with the slightly older Kaushik, who is a lonely and aloof teenager. She reveals both his literal and metaphorical hunger as she describes his habit of eating great quantities of grapes and apples, both fruits which she herself did not eat at the time (Lahiri 2009, 240). Throughout this piece, Kaushik's mother—who is secretly battling breast cancer, and who dies by the end of this first story—tries very hard to maintain the strength to remain involved in preparing the food he loves. When Hema's mother prepares a big pot of khichuri, Kaushik's mother insists on helping, and she makes her eagerly anticipated English trifle for him as well (Lahiri 2009, 247). Hema tries it herself and doesn't care for it, but notices that he "devoured bowl after bowl; your mother finally put it away, fearing that you would get a stomachache" (Lahiri 2009, 248). We thus see two important factors that set up the way food is involved in the second and third parts of this story. For Hema, observing Kaushik's eating habits becomes part of her close attention to him and to her "education" in the unfamiliar; we will see her return to this in the third story, which alternates between her and his narrative viewpoint. And for Kaushik, we understand how his complicated feelings about food in the second story (which is told from his point of view when he is a college student, several years after his mother's death) have been influenced by his feelings of connection to his mother and his grief over losing her.

This second story begins when Kaushik returns to the home of his father, who has married a woman named Chitra with two young daughters and who has recently brought his new wife and her children to live with him in the United States Kaushik is bemused by Chitra's behavior as a traditional Indian housewife and hostess, as she sets out an elaborate meal for him: "I was no longer accustomed to Indian food. At school I ate in the cafeteria, and during my time at home after my mother's death my father and I either went out or picked up pizzas" (Lahiri 2009, 259–60). He is torn between his hunger and his discomfort: "My mouth watered, in spite of my reluctance to eat, and I was suddenly grateful for the vast amount of food in front of me . . . [but] the arrangement of the bowls . . . felt too formal" (Lahiri 2009, 261). And it is through this act of attempting to serve him, especially when he makes a move for the kitchen and Chitra immediately offers to get him whatever he needs, that Kaushik begins to show his resentment for the woman who has replaced his dead mother: "I was suddenly sickened by her, by the sight of her standing in our kitchen" (Lahiri 2009, 263).

Interestingly, as Kaushik thinks about his mother's illness and eventual death, he expresses his memories in terms of the nurse, Mrs. Gharibian, who took care of her at the end of her life, and the food that she prepared for them:

> She would bring Tupperware containers full of lamb turnovers and stuffed grape leaves, food that now reminds me of my mother dying, putting them in the refrigerator for my father and me to eat, also stocking the house with milk and bread without being asked. Normally she left in the evenings, but for two weeks she spent the nights with us, administering morphine injections and emptying the bedpans, making notes in a little cloth book that looked as if it ought to contain recipes. Something about her quietly optimistic manner made me believe that Mrs. Gharibian had the power to sustain my mother, not to cure her but to keep her alive indefinitely. (Lahiri 2009, 267)

He is moved by others' attempts to nurture and nourish him, yet he also feels deeply ambivalent because he harbors such deep feelings of grief and loss. This becomes even clearer in the sequence of events that happens with Chitra's daughters, as he himself both acts as nurturer and eventually withdraws in anger (as he will do again with Hema in the third story). When Chitra offers Kaushik tea in the morning and he says that he will get coffee at Dunkin Donuts instead, he explains what a donut is, and later brings Rupa and Piu, the daughters, there with him, where they are fascinated by the selection. Not knowing which kind to pick, they choose Boston Cream when he says it's his favorite, and he watches them as they devour the doughnuts to the last bite (Lahiri 2009, 272). After he sends them back over to the counter to pick out which donuts they want to bring their mother, he admonishes them for simply pointing to their selections (since they are too shy to speak to the cashier). Kaushik feels some empathy for them as he recalls his own alienation and fear when he first arrived in the United States, and there is some potential for connection here. However, when he discovers that Rupa and Piu have been rifling through the hidden box of photos that he has kept of his mother, he explodes in anger and flees, undertaking an odyssey along the New England coast, unable to deal with the profound sense of rage and sorrow at his mother's death that the episode has created for him.

At the end of this story, Kaushik returns to images of food, this time in his description of the meals that he has in various diners in the fishing villages. Here, we witness his attempt to heal by creating new rituals for himself, and by finding solace even in bad food: "When I think of it I still savor the taste of diner coffee that was at once bitter and insipid, the waffles drowned in syrup, the gummy chowder and greasy eggs, as if no other food had nourished me before then" (Lahiri 2009, 290). In other words, he is only able to move past his grief by learning to eat on his own, and to seek sustenance through sources that he does not identify with his mother, his culture, or his past. He clearly still craves being fed, being nurtured, but he actively substitutes nostalgia for his childhood with a later nostalgia for the food he associates with this period of rebellion and independence.

The third "Hema and Kaushik" story, which alternates their points of view in third-person limited narration, focuses on the two characters years later when they finally reunite. It begins with Hema, who is now an academic trying to focus on her classical studies work while in Rome. She keeps returning to the same restaurant for her meals there because each time that she tried a different spot, the food was underwhelming to her or she was embarrassed by her poor command of Italian (Lahiri 2009, 295). As she recalls her earlier travels with Julian, her ex-boyfriend who was married to another woman while she was seeing him, she thinks of the hotel breakfasts that they would eat together; her simultaneous attraction and repulsion in the relationship seems to be connected to the food imagery she conjures up here as she remembers the birds that would gather at their feet during their breakfasts of ricotta and mortadella and salami: "She had been disconcerted by those salty, fleshy meats so early in the day, yet never able to resist them" (Lahiri 2009, 296).

After Hema and Kaushik find one another again at a dinner party hosted by a mutual friend, they become lovers. Yet the act of eating for them is described in very particular, streamlined ways, as if all of their sexual energy is channeled into their physical passion for one another rather than being deflected onto food. When Hema spends the night at Kaushik's apartment, she discovers that there's no food in his refrigerator except for salted biscotti and mineral water. They take pleasure in staying together at a convent in Volterra where the "food was plainer, bowls of ribollita, bread without salt, bittersweet hot chocolate in the afternoons. As they ate their meals . . . they, too, felt fortified, tranquil, much like the town" (Lahiri 2009, 319). And when they have lunch in a restaurant on the Piazza del Priori, again, the food is sensual but simple: "bruschetta with black cabbage, soft pappardelle flecked with wild boar" (Lahiri 2009, 320).

The tragedy of the story is that despite their strong feelings for one another, both Hema and Kaushik are stubborn about not wanting to give up their solo careers. Hema ends up agreeing to the arranged marriage that her family had set up for her, and Kaushik travels to a resort north of Khao Lak in Thailand, where (unbeknownst to him) the tsunami is about to arrive and end his life. Strikingly, Kaushik's quick immersion in a routine of meals at the resort hearkens back to his attempts to self-comfort at the New England diners on the coast (another waterfront) in the second story, and it also brings him back to his childhood memories of the food that he would eat when his mother was still alive:

> [A]lready he felt drugged by the routine: getting out of bed, eating fruit and sticky rolls for breakfast . . . The food reminded him a little of his childhood: steaming rice, dense brown and yellow curries, whole red and green chilies floating in sauce. Normally he harbored no nostalgia for the particular elements of his upbringing, adapting to so many cuisines throughout his adult life. But this food caused him to feel strangely sentimental. (Lahiri 2009, 325)

When he first arrives in Thailand, Kaushik is consumed with anger at Hema, but his feelings turn rapidly into longing for her (though he is too stubborn or too passive to contact her). He feels so strongly for Hema in part because she was a part of his past, and knew his mother, and understands him in a way that other women have not. In this sense, since he is unable to act upon his desire for the relationship to have lasted, he effectively conflates the loss of his mother and the loss of Hema with the feelings of nostalgia that he gets from eating the curries. When the tsunami comes, he is out on a boat ride and has just submerged himself in the water to swim, enjoying its womblike warmth, never knowing what hit him. Heidi Elizabeth Bollinger looks at the way this moment is prefigured several times earlier in the linked stories; she describes Lahiri's "profoundly haunting use of disaster as endpoint" (Bollinger 2014, 502).

As for Hema—who picks up the concluding narrative viewpoint of this last story, but switches from third person limited to first person—she is back in India, shopping for wedding garments (for the arranged marriage) with her mother and two aunts, and had been "oblivious" all day to the news of the tsunami. She remarks that they had spent hours that afternoon "drinking Cokes and eating mutton rolls . . . But the whole time

I was thinking of you, fearful of the mistake I was making. I was still slightly jet-lagged, hungry for meals we were used to eating together, for the taste of good coffee and wine" (Lahiri 2009, 331). Her consumption of the Cokes and mutton rolls marks the return to American/Indian food tourist food culture. Like Kaushik, her focus on food marks a semi-indirect way of acknowledging a longing for the past that they had together: she longs for the simpler and yet more sophisticated food and drink they shared because it is too painful for her to consider directing that longing into an attempt to recontact him. In the closing lines of the story, she has heard of Kaushik's fate, has gotten married, and is now pregnant: a more contrived narrative would have had it turn out that the baby is Kaushik's. Instead, Hema's final words pointing out that this is *not* the case underscore the heartbreaking nature of the story: "It might have been your child but this was not the case. We had been careful, and you had left nothing behind" (Lahiri 2009, 333).

In Shelby Silas's play *Calcutta Kosher*, Mozelle, a dying matriarch, attempts to conduct a dinner party attended by her estranged daughters; in the process, we find out about some of the hidden secrets of her past. The discussion that follows examines Silas's play as a food narrative, with an emphasis on how the portrayal of food/eating/cooking/hunger underscores not only the generational conflicts within the play, but also the clashes that occur involving caste, ethnicity, and religion. Moreover, the inclusion of recipes in the playscript (an unusual choice) sets up a complex conversation between Silas and her audience/readers.

In order to make sense of this play, a little bit of background about Jewish-Indian identity is helpful. With the exception of Desai's 1988 novel *Baumgartner's Bombay*, very little literary attention has been paid to the fascinating intercultural implications of the presence of Jews in India. A spice trader created the first Baghdadi Jewish settlement in Calcutta in 1798, and for hundreds of years, there were large Jewish communities there as well as in Bombay (now Mumbai) and Cochin. What many readers may not know, though, is that there is an entire cuisine of Jewish-Indian (or Indian-Jewish) food that both literally and symbolically reflects a long history of this specific cultural fusion. In an August 2006 essay in the *London Times*, Zaki Cooper—whose grandmother was part of the Indian-Jewish community in Calcutta—uses the news of Indian Jews being outraged by a restaurant in Mumbai that was decorated with Nazi paraphernalia as the springboard for her own efforts to provide an account of this community. She writes:

> More surprising for many people was the news that India has a Jewish community at all. Being a descendant of that community I am used to this surprise. Visitors to my grandmother on festive days are surprised by the scents of curry which fill the home instead of roast chicken,

lockshen and pickled herring. What smells like an experiment in cross-cultural affairs is in fact a typical scene in a Jewish household from India. (Cooper 2006, 74)

Mavis Hyman's *Indian-Jewish Cooking*, while ostensibly a cookbook, actually provides a very detailed illustrated account of what makes this cultural group and this cuisine entirely unique. Hyman, who was born in Calcutta of Iraqi-Jewish parents, traces her roots on her mother's side to the Jews who settled in Calcutta over two hundred years ago; though she emigrated to Great Britain, she wanted to preserve the legacy of this community, particularly given the "gradual but almost complete disintegration of the Jewish community in Calcutta" (Hyman 1992, 15). To develop the recipes, she spent years consulting with Indian Jews in Bombay (Mumbai), Calcutta, and Cochin; many of the cooks from whom she learned techniques were of her mother's generation and have subsequently passed away. The book, then, is significant not just as a culinary resource, but also as a sort of cultural document that includes hand-illustrated depictions of tools and spices.

Silas's play was inspired by Hyman's book as well as by Silas's own family history (she was born in Calcutta and grew up in North London). *Calcutta Kosher* was first produced by the Kali Theatre Company at Southwark Playhouse in 2004, followed by a very successful run in Stratford. It received somewhat mixed reviews from the British press: some, like Benedict Nightingale in the *London Times* and Nick Curtis in the *Evening Standard*, criticized the lack of plot, and Mike Parker of the *Morning Star* had issues with the direction of the Stratford production. Others, though, were impressed with Silas's attention to a marginalized cultural community. Michael Billington of the *Guardian* wrote that the play "emerges as an elegiac hymn to a disappearing world" and said that the "emphasis on reconciliation and harmony also lends it an unusual sweetness of temper" (Billington 2004, 26). Like many reviewers, John Peter of the *London Sunday Times* did not know that there was a Jewish-Indian community in Calcutta, and remarked, "The theatre does teach you things." He goes on to offer a more generous assessment of the play than some of his peers:

> This is a play about belonging. Where is home? What is home? . . . [W]ho decides whether you belong or not? And if you don't belong, who are you? . . . This is a wise, compassionate, moving play, studded with sharp but melancholy jokes and acted with hard but touching emotional intelligence: a gem that glows in the dark. (Peter 2004, 24)

Like Mavis Hyman in *Indian-Jewish Cooking*, Silas is interested in telling the story of a rapidly vanishing group; in her introduction to the piece, she points out that "It is probably easier to say what Indian Jews are not, rather than what they are," emphasizing that they are not Ashkenazi (Eastern European) Jews, nor are they "part of the Raj, nor Anglo Indians. They are a culture unique both to India and to international

Jewry" (Silas 2004, n.p.). At the time she was writing this introduction, she says, there were no more than thirty Indian Jews remaining in Calcutta.

The opening stage set gives us the immediate contrast between the past and the present, as we see both old family furniture (*morahs*) in Mozelle the matriarch's Calcutta house as well as a new Apple laptop. Dietary and religious restrictions are mentioned almost immediately as Mozelle remarks to Maki, her young caregiver (who we find out is her daughter by another man), that she has never had pork, since she is Jewish and it is "forbidden" (Silas 2004, 20). As Mozelle's daughter Esther shows up, we also see that Mozelle has an old-school servant, Siddique, about whom we will learn more later but who, in the opening scenes, is largely unacknowledged by the other characters. When Mozelle says they should think about dinner and Esther says that food is the last thing on her mind—she is concerned because Mozelle has had a heart attack—Mozelle responds, "You must always think about food" (Silas 2004, 26) and goes on to name her favorite dishes. Esther tells Mozelle that she doesn't make "their" food at home because her children are fussy eaters and Peter, her husband, who is an Ashkenazi (Eastern European) Jew, doesn't think it's plain enough. Mozelle doesn't drop the subject just yet, though:

MOZELLE: Does he like chicken soup?

ESTHER: Sometimes.

MOZELLE: You should make him Pish Posh.

ESTHER: He calls it baby food.

MOZELLE: I suppose he likes egg and chips? Sunny side up.

ESTHER: Not always.

MOZELLE: Tomato sauce?

ESTHER: Occasionally.

MOZELLE: It is the devil's blood.

ESTHER: It's not that bad.

MOZELLE: Fish balls?

ESTHER: Of course.

MOZELLE: I didn't know fish had them. (MOZELLE *laughs to herself.*) (Silas 2004, 26)

The conversation is revealing in several respects. Mozelle clearly defines others according to their tastes in food, and her scrutiny of Peter's eating habits attempts to mark him as Jewish (the chicken soup, the gefilte fish) but also belies her contempt for his potentially British preferences (eggs and chips, ketchup). Her comments before and after this conversation about Esther's weight gain suggest that for her, food is both an apparatus for judgment and a marker of distinct cultural and religious status. She even returns shortly after this to the earlier subject of pigs, asking Esther suspiciously whether she or Peter eats pig and reminding her that it's not kosher. Esther, though, feels resistant to Mozelle's attempts to assert her matriarchal status, confiding to Maki that she spent so much time in boarding school and with aunts in London that the house doesn't even really feel like her home.

After Mozelle's other daughter, Silvie—who is a bit of a prima donna—arrives, we see Siddique, the servant, enter with two bowls of food for Mozelle: one is Mahmoosa, which is a dish made of eggs, potatoes, onions, and spices, and the other is Chukla Bukla, which is vegetables pickled in vinegar. When Esther says that she thought they were having dinner later, Maki explains that Mozelle eats "little and often"; Silvie takes the spoon away and attempts to feed her mother, who refuses to eat until Siddique resumes feeding her (Silas 2004, 42). Maki and Siddique have a conversation in Hindustani (which the other characters don't understand) about how he'll go start the potatoes for the dinner party, and when she describes the dishes they'll be having, Silvie expresses some surprise that Maki knows "the art of Indian-Jewish cooking" (Silas 2004, 45), and Maki explains that she learned it from Siddique: "Ma never cooked. But she said it should be preserved and the tradition should be kept" (Silas 2004, 45); meanwhile, Silvie, who has clearly distanced herself from these traditions, asks if they can also have a salad. Strikingly, then, the task of maintaining the cultural past has fallen to the more marginalized members of the household, while the two elder daughters, both more assimilated into colonialist practices, express their ambivalence. This also becomes the key to understanding the greater tensions in the play that are beginning to surface between Maki, the mother's so-called "love child," and Esther and Silvie, who on some level resent her presence and fail to understand her significance in the household.

The assimilated daughters' ambivalence about traditional food is further complicated by the revelation that it was actually a food item that supported their family: Mozelle comments that they should go see the new owner of her late husband's (Esther and Silvie's father) pickle factory: "How that man has ruined it. We made pickles and we were proud of them" (Silas 2004, 53). When Silvie comments disdainfully, Mozelle admonishes her that they were only able to afford to send her to school in England because of pickles: "The very best. Lime, mango, brinjal. I can still taste it" (Silas 2004, 53), to which Silvie responds that her husband hates pickles and finds them "too hot and spicy" (Silas 2004, 53), again showing the generational and cultural gap present here. Mozelle even confides to Maki that she wishes Esther had married Nathan, whose father's business was exporting pickles from her husband's factory.

It is through the combination of food and Jewish ritual that the tensions between Mozelle and her two eldest daughters explodes at the end of Act One. As Maki lays out the bread and wine to be blessed for the Jewish Sabbath, Silvie asks why Maki is the one chosen to do the blessing, and Mozelle finally admits that not only is Maki Jewish, but that she is also really her mother. Esther and Silvie react with anger—Esther refuses to take the bread that Maki has just blessed—but the scene comes to an abrupt end when Mozelle begins choking on the bread. As the daughters watch over Mozelle in the beginning of the second act, Silvie eats little pieces of bread but also chides herself for doing so; it's striking that Mozelle resumes her alert motherly stance almost immediately when she sees Silvie pushing the bread away and says that they need to have food brought to them. Silvie says, "I'm not hungry hungry," a qualifier that does not suit Mozelle, who commands, "You will eat" (Silas 2004, 71). And when Siddique brings the food, Silvie admits that she "could manage a little something" (Silas 2004, 74). When Mozelle starts to choke again—this time because of the hot chilis in the Chukla Bukla pickles— Esther and Maki both attempt to hand her a glass of water at the same time, but Esther lets go and allows Maki to give it to her. We see in these two sequences, then, that if there is any possibility for eventual forgiveness and community here, despite the elder daughters' resistance, it may come about through the act of sharing a meal.

Mozelle reveals more about her backstory as the dinner continues, telling her eldest daughters that their father was actually supposed to marry her sister Maisie, who was actually in love with a Hindu boy— which was forbidden—and subsequently withdrew from the world. She admits that Maisie knew and understood about the secret love she harbored for Ravi, Maki's father, and Esther and Silvie take out their shock and anger about this revelation by once again turning on Maki for keeping secrets. Maki stands up to them, though, asking them how it felt to have her and Siddique—since they assumed she was a servant like him— washing their dishes, ironing their clothes, and cooking their food. We see the deeply ingrained class and caste biases of the elder daughters in a comical moment, right after they have made their assumption that Siddique doesn't speak English, when he casually answers Silvie's sarcastic "What do you think, Siddique?" regarding whether the Calcutta synagogues should be shipped to museums with "Bad idea" (Silas 2004, 84).

Unlike Esther, though, Silvie—despite all of her sarcasm—seems more willing to accept Maki as a sister and to accept that their mother loved another man besides their father. As they talk, the stage directions indicate that despite her earlier ambivalence about eating, she piles her plate with food and eats it. She says:

> I should learn to make this. We could have a family cookbook. The three sisters Indian Jewish Cook Book. All your family favourites and more. You know Siddique never taught us how to cook. We had servants for that. (Silas 2004, 87)

On the one hand, her acknowledgment of "three" sisters, which therefore includes Maki, is huge. On the other hand, as they go on to discuss Siddique, we see how little Silvie really knows about him, as Maki has to explain the choices he has made about why and how he serves the family.

As Mozelle talks to the daughters about her imminent death—which she jokingly calls "going to the great pickle factory in the sky" (Silas 2004, 89)—she urges upon them the importance of preserving their Jewish community's food, culture, and identity, adding a bit later that she has made arrangements in her will for helping to preserve the Calcutta synagogues. (And Zaki Cooper's essay also mentions these "ornate and beautiful" synagogues, many of which still receive attention from visitors [Cooper 2006, 74].) Mozelle asks to be dressed in her wedding outfit from the 1950s and begins to pray in Hebrew as Maki reveals that earlier, Mozelle bribed the doctor not to come back. The play ends with a shift from Hebrew to Hindustani as Maki repeats a song that Mozelle sang to her earlier and which translates as "Sleep sleep baby sleep sleep. Butter bread sugar. Butter bread finished. Small baby slept" (Silas 2004, 62). In a powerful moment, Silvie joins Maki in singing the song, and as the lights fade, Siddique sings the song alone. Not only is it powerful to see this return to simple images of food and nourishing, but the sequence also indicates the change in Silvie as she takes part in the song and therefore acknowledges that she is honoring the connection her mother had to Maki and Siddique and to her mother's buried past.

At the end of the published version of the play, Silas includes recipes for four of the dishes that the characters eat during the play itself: Mahmoosa, which is made from eggs, potatoes, and spices; Aloomakallas, which are potatoes with a golden crust; Chittarnee, which is a sweet and sour chicken curry; and Chukla Bukla, or pickled vegetable. The recipes are punctuated with encouraging comments: "Allow two hours for this recipe. It's worth it!"; "Good luck!"; "Simply delicious" (Silas 2004, 105, 108). I want to close with some attention to the gesture of including these recipes, for two reasons. In production, to whatever extent a director and designer choose to replicate the actual cooking and serving of these dishes on stage, the permeation of the theater with the scents of spices like turmeric, garlic, ginger, and coriander has a visceral impact upon the audience: we may not be sharing these dishes with Mozelle and her daughters, but we take them in on a primal level. And for readers of the play script, the recipes are a significant expansion of the boundaries of the text as we are invited—and as I pointed out, warmly encouraged—to participate in the preservation of cultural memory by becoming authors of our own versions of these dishes. For Silas's characters, as for Desai's and Lahiri's, there is no easy recipe, no true formula, for reaching the point where this voluntary act of preservation happens: ultimately, though, to embrace the past entails an acknowledgment of one's hungers, even when doing so is inordinately painful.

FOUR

Feeding the Audience

Food, Feminism, and Performance Art

At what point, then, does the satisfaction of one's hunger become a type of performance? One spring morning not too many years ago, in the midst of the commuter rush on the #6 train in New York City, I watched a man unwrap (slowly, lovingly) the various parts of his breakfast (Egg McMuffin, hash browns in styrofoam container, coffee with cream and sugar) and proceed—wholly oblivious to the crowd, the noise, the dirt of the subway car—to eat his food, slurping his coffee and spilling Egg McMuffin crumbs onto his business suit, absorbed in his meal to the point of being unaware that the eyes of every commuter in that subway car were upon him.

In my women's studies courses, when we talk about food, I ask the women in the room if they have ever felt self-conscious eating in public. Invariably, several of them recount stories of "first dates" during which they scanned the menu for something that would be easy to eat inconspicuously, picking a salad or chicken breast for fear that devouring a plate of spaghetti would expose an overeager appetite and would risk stains and spills and messiness; only later, still hungry and safely away from the judging eye across the table, would they open the refrigerator and stuff themselves with cold pizza, ice cream straight from the carton, anything deliciously gooey and sloppy.

It strikes me that in both of these cases, eating becomes the site of a public performance: an unself-conscious one for the man on the subway, and the opposite for the woman in the restaurant. Our boundaries between the public and the private are challenged at the moments when the primal act of feeding, having entered the realm of culture, become spec(tac)ular. Perhaps part of the appeal, for some, of watching county

73

fair eating contests has been the opportunity to indulge vicariously, or voyeuristically, in a kind of obscene excess (similar to that which one can witness in porn films?); watching, or perhaps also engaging in, an orgy of public eating is simultaneously repulsive and gratifying in its temporary violation of cultural sanctions against appetite, sloppiness, and extreme consumption.

In postmodern American culture, the spectacle of consumption has extended to the preparation of food itself as a form of performance; one need only think of Benihana and sushi bar chefs, supermarket food demonstrators, and TV cooking shows as examples of the theatricalization of appetite—and, I would argue, the transference of gratification from the visceral to the visual. In the case of the "live" chefs and food demonstrators, one may be invited to partake of what has been prepared, but TV cooking shows offer the possibility of satisfying and denying the appetite at the same time. In perhaps the most vicarious forms of consumption, the spectacle itself is stripped of visible human agency: commercials and magazine covers or advertisements (and sometimes, Instagram and other social media photos with filters) offer food that—like performers themselves, with makeup and coiffure and lighting assistance—has been "stylized," dressed up and staged like *Playboy* centerfolds for our visual projections of consumerist fantasies. Rosalind Coward went so far as to call such photographs "food pornography" (Coward 1985, 101–6) and "food porn" later became a common term to describe such images. Coward suggests that the images' appeal to the forbidden, their relation to female servitude and objectification, and their repression of the processes of production resemble the aesthetic and ideological practices of the photos in soft-core mainstream centerfold pictures. As Jeremy MacClancy puts it, "Cropped close-ups may show a fat piece of gilded chicken, a larger-than-life cream tart with a hyper-real texture, or a slice of sponge cake, its dark chocolate filling threatening to ooze over the edge. Either way the message is not understated, but shouted: 'Eat me! Eat me!'" (MacClancy 1992, 141). (For more on the male gaze and its role in objectification, see Berger 1972, 45–64, and Mulvey 1995.)

All of this goes a long way toward explaining why, in the theater, the performance of eating or preparing food is a subject of fascination. Two well-known playwrights for whom the "staging" of food figures repeatedly are Sam Shepard and Tina Howe. Shepard's plays featured everything from pouring milk into a bowl of Rice Krispies over a character's hand (*Forensic and the Navigators*) to frying bacon and boiling artichokes on stage (*Curse of the Starving Class*) to having characters carry in piles of corn and carrots (*Buried Child*) to making real toast in dozens of toasters that a character has stolen throughout the neighborhood and plugged in to impress his brother (*True West*). (For further discussion of the role of food and other objects in Shepard's work, see chap. 3 in Garner 1994.) Howe's work is concerned with more explicitly "female" images associating cooking and eating with problems of sexuality and creativity. While this exists mostly in narrative form in *Painting Churches*, *The Art of Dining* takes place in a restaurant where we see food being cooked and eaten, and Howe's later play *One Shoe Off* revolves around a dinner party gone haywire. (For further discussion of the role of food in Howe's work, see Backes 1989, 41–60.) Both Shepard and Howe were aware of the spectacle inherent in the theatrical presentation of food and excess, as well as the pleasure of juxtaposing the corporeal/ tangible (and "smellable") realm of real food with the fictionalized/vicarious/untouchable realm of staged performance.

Part of the appeal of food in narrative drama, then, is simply the novelty of its "realness" when encountered in a medium that we are aware is *not* "real"; the audience of Shepard's *Curse of the Starving Class*, for instance, can smell the bacon actually cooking in a pan at the beginning of the play—a field of experience not available to them as film or television spectators. Performance art, though, goes one step further. Since performance art itself challenges the boundaries between the "lived" and the "performed," food in works of performance art—though usually still "framed" by the parameters of a designation as a performance "piece," and still (again, usually) presented before "consumers," or spectators—is somewhat liberated from its role as a novel mode of disrupting the fictional/narrative milieu.[1] In its foregrounding of the gendered/sexual desiring body, its conflations of and transgressions of private and public spaces, its connections with ritual, its paradoxical impermanence and corporeality, and its challenging of a consuming and consumerist audience, performance art becomes a site for theorizing the relationships between food and the spec(tac)ular—and our "eating culture," correspondingly, becomes terrain for better exploring the pleasures and possibilities of performance art. This chapter describes precursors to more recent food "performances," then focuses on several women performance artists, including Karen Finley, for whom the preparation, consumption, or reappropriation of food addresses the relationships of eating, gendered bodies, and public spaces.

A fascinating precursor to contemporary performance art's interest in relationships between food and the body is the *lazzi* of the Commedia dell'Arte which flourished in Europe between 1550 and 1750. *Lazzi* were stock comic routines, often involving sexual, scatological, and violent slapstick, employed repeatedly in the *commedia* as a way of generating guaranteed laughter. It is possible to argue that despite their insertion into essentially narrative frameworks, the *lazzi*—in their emphasis on the body, their interplay with the audience, and their disruption of or disregard for the play's "plot"—were a version of popular performance art. In Mel Gordon's *lazzi* from this era, an entire section is devoted to routines involving food. As Gordon points out, many of the *lazzi* drew upon an infantile fascination with seeking food, consuming enormous quantities of it or making a mess with it, and calling attention to the processes of excretion. I am particularly interested in the *lazzi* that involved the conflation of food and the body to the point that the body *becomes* food. In the "Lazzo of Being Brained," for instance, Arlecchino receives a blow on the head that is so strong that his "brains begin to spurt out." In response, "afraid that he will lose his intelligence, Arlecchino sits and feasts on his brains" (Gordon 1983, 23). And the "Lazzo of Eating Oneself" proceeds as follows: "Famished, Arlecchino can find nothing to eat but himself. Starting with his feet and working up to his knees, thighs, and upper torso, Arlecchino devours himself" (Gordon 1983, 23).

The transgressive (cannibalistic, masturbatory) quality of this act, as well as the absurd impossibility of the performer consuming himself (how would this be staged?) calls attention to the way that performance forces us to make leaps of the imagination; there is a beautifully Escherian (il)logic to what Arlecchino is doing. In a manner that calls to mind the performance pieces of Karen Finley, whose works will be discussed shortly, Arlecchino's action mirrors and parodies the spectators' appetite for "devouring" the performer's body. As with the *lazzi*, performance art has a predilection for taking such metaphors of consumption—always to some degree present in the theater—and pushing them toward a literalization, or embodiment, that (in the playful manner of much postmodern art) can be both serious and ludicrous at the same time.

The Futurists and Surrealists, too, staged playful events with food that can be considered early versions of performance art. In Russia in 1913 and 1914, Natalia Goncharova, Vladimir Larionov, Vladimir Mayakofsky, and the Burliuk brothers made a film, *Drama in Cabaret No. 13*, about their activity of walking in the streets with flowers and vegetables in their arms, radishes in their buttonholes, and algebraic symbols painted on their faces (Henri 1974, 14). In Italy, the food "events" of Marinetti and his followers have been well documented (see Marinetti 1989 for a description of these activities). Salvador Dalí gave a lecture in London in 1936 with a loaf of French bread strapped to a helmet; in *The Secret Life of Salvador Dalí*, he describes his idea of making giant loaves of bread appear suddenly in conspicuous public places in Paris and other European cities. Dalí claims that the effect would be one of "collective hysteria," and the spectacle would thus become "the point of departure from which . . . one could subsequently try to ruin . . . systematically the logical meaning of all the mechanisms of the rational practical world" (qtd. in Henri 1974, 24).

As performance art began to take on its own meanings distinct from visual art, several "environmental" artists in the early 1960s through the mid-1970s began to experiment with creating interactive environments involving the preparation, serving, consumption, and sometimes decomposition of food. Daniel Spoerri (*Restaurant Spoerri*) in Dusseldorf and Les

Levine (*Levine's Restaurant*) in New York set up actual restaurants; their "art" was the event of diners entering the space, discussing and consuming the food, and paying for it (Henri 1974, 41; for a description of Spoerri's other works involving food, see Henri 1974, 146, 156). In a sense, Spoerri and Levine enacted a parody of the manner in which other, more traditional works of art are "consumed" by spectators who enter a gallery and "devour" the paintings; the impermanence of both the environment and the food in it called attention to the sense (also prevalent in Allan Kaprow's "Happenings," another performance art precursor that often involved food) that an artwork could be transitory and experiential, evolving only in its moments of reception.

Merret Oppenheim, one of the few women French Surrealists, created a piece entitled *Spring Feast* for the Tenth Surrealist Exhibition of 1959. In it, a golden-faced woman (a real one in the private viewing of the piece) was stretched out on a long dinner table, her body covered with fruit, and surrounded by men (again, real ones at the private viewing) sitting at the table, poised to consume her (Henri 1974, 60). In many ways, Oppenheim's creation anticipated those of the women performance artists whose works emerged a decade or so later. Perhaps because of the obvious cultural connections between food and the female body as object for consumption, women performance artists in particular have used their work to call attention to, and sometimes to parody, these connections. (For further discussion of the "consumable" female body, see Coward 1985 and Adams 1990.) Sue-Ellen Case points out that doing so risks posing a "biologistic" model of female oppression that may, according to materialist feminists, simply participate in a mythologizing and universalizing of the female body at the expense of more socially and politically motivated critiques of such oppression. She cites Judy Chicago's "Dinner Party" as an example of "the formal influence of such biologistic thinking" (Case 1988, 55–56; for an artist's point of view, see Chicago 1977). Although Case's point is well taken, I would argue that most of the women performance artists that I am about to describe, though sometimes essentialist in their tendency to privilege one female body (the performer's) as "representative" of "the female body," do incorporate a greater degree of materialist critique into the works than Case is willing to give them credit for having done.[2] Indeed, I think that by the specific strategies these artists use to communicate with (and sometimes to confront) their *audiences*, they question and politicize issues of representation; further, since food itself is a cultural commodity, its use moves their pieces beyond the biologistic and into the realm of *material* examinations of consumerism in its various forms (as mentioned above).[3]

Carolee Schneeman's *Meat Joy* (1964) celebrated—and to some degree eroticized—the associations between genital sexuality and meat as performers rolled nude on the floor in a display of orgiastic pleasure, covering themselves with shreds of paper, paint, sausages, fish, and chicken (see Birringer 1993, 44). A series of photographs by Suzanne Lacy entitled *The Anatomy Lesson* (1973–1976) included a sequence of Lacy consuming various parts of a chicken (*Wing, Arm, Breast Leg*) and another of her as a crazed, wild-eyed Julia Child explaining *Where the Meat Comes From* by wielding her knife at a lamb carcass (see Roth 1988, 56). In her early works, Linda Montano went from exhibiting chickens as "living sculptures" in galleries to dressing up as "Chicken Woman" (1971) and displaying herself in public places, thus mocking the connections between her own gender and her status as "food" or consumable object (see Montano 1981, 51). Schneeman, Lacy, and Montano, like several other women performance artists, take on the "biologistic" model by deconstructing what Carol Adams calls the "texts of meat." According to Adams, the "patriarchal nature of our meat-advocating cultural discourse" enforces social attitudes of reverence toward meat as a repository of signification, a "meaningful" food. Adams argues that this overwhelming sense of meat as an embodiment of "coherence" comes from "patriarchal attitudes including the idea that the end justifies the means, that the objectification of other beings is a necessary part of life, and that violence can and should be masked" (Adams 1990, 14). All of these cultural assumptions, in Adams's view, underly the "sexual politics of meat." Women performance artists who take on a critique of the sexual politics of meat may, on one level, be employing a "biologistic" model in Case's sense, given that the subject matter is the very material taken into their bodies; on the other hand, the "texts of meat" are also materialist texts about the gendering of consumption and consumerism. While such pieces as *Meat Joy* foregrounded ritual, others—like Montano's Chicken Woman, or Nina Sobell's video performance *Baby Chicky* (1981)—drew upon the ironies of the woman-meat image to create a more critical and materialist view. In *Baby Chicky*, the artist appeared nude with a raw chicken on her head and another cradled in her arms. Sobell's text reinforces the sense that little girls grow up prepared to become (and to see themselves as) pieces of meat:

> Once upon a time there was a little girl whose job it was to clean and season the Friday Night Chicken and put it in the oven. She stood on a stool so she could reach down into the sink to wash and shower the chicken with cool, clean water. When she held the chicken up it started to dance on the floor of the sink while the little girl sang. When they were finished playing and the chicken was sleepy she put it into the bedpan and into the oven. If the little girl was bad, or her mommy thought she was, she would pick up the little girl and say, "One, two, three, into the oven you go," and the little girl would say, "Hey, Ma, I might be bad but I ain't chicken." (Sobell 1981, 78)

The domestic space of the kitchen is the realm of the private, a realm most often associated with the female (I had a landlord who said to me, only half-jokingly, "A woman's place is in the oven"). The public space of performance allows women artists to interrogate the boundaries between the private and the public; as I mentioned at the beginning of this essay, entering the territory of public space through food can be a transgressive or defiant act, and some women performance artists have chosen to focus on—sometimes to literalize—the crossing of those boundaries. Nancy Barber, for instance, chose to "make visible" the domestic sphere by showing videos of people cooking in their homes on a local cable television channel (Montano 1981, 47). As a reversal that brought the domestic into theatrical space, in Allison Knowles's "concert" piece *Make a Salad* (first performed by the Fluxus Group in Denmark in 1962, and repeated many times since then), an audience enters a concert hall, expecting a musical performance, but the "music" turns out to be the sounds and rhythms of the performers chopping carrots, tearing lettuce, and so forth, to make a huge salad for the audience to help consume (Montano 1981, 46). In Barbara Smith's *Feed Me* (1973), the artist arranged a private room in a gallery where she sat nude, surrounded by items of comfort and nurturing such as soft pillows and a mattress and rug, food, incense, candles, wine, scented oils, and so forth; visitors were invited to enter the space individually to interact with her. As Jeanie Forte points out, although the piece was criticized for furthering audience voyeurism, the crucial distinction is that Smith was emphasizing her own pleasure (Forte points out that the piece was entitled *"Feed Me,"* not "let me feed you," and therefore Smith did not simply make herself into a kind of "food" for the audience to consume [Forte 1992, 257]).

Performance artist Bonnie Sherk defied the boundaries of the public and the private even more overtly in a piece entitled *Public Lunch* (1971), which was the culmination of a series of performances in various locations entitled *Sitting Still*. Sherk arranged herself as an "exhibit" in the lions' house at the San Francisco Zoo so that she became, in effect, another "animal" on display for the spectators walking by. At feeding time, just when the lions were being thrown their raw, red hunks of meat, Sherk (dressed in formal wear) had an elegant catered lunch delivered to her, and ate it at a small, formally arranged table in her cage next to the lions' cage. The piece is interesting in several respects in addition to the clearly parodic (or "ethical") statement it makes about zoos and their purposes. Sherk comments, "It was about analogies and being an object on view" (Montano 1981, 50). By timing her meal to coincide with the lions', Sherk interrogates the differences between "civilized" and "primitive" rituals of eating, suggesting perhaps that the trappings of civilization (the silverware, tablecloth, etc.) are merely devices for deluding ourselves into thinking that our feeding does not serve the same primal purpose as it does for the lions tearing apart their raw meat in their cage.

Sherk's performance—which could be interpreted as a feminist response to Kafka's story "A Hunger Artist"—challenges the voyeuristic desire of the passersby (her audience) to *watch* her in the zoo, particularly while she is engaged in the act of eating.[4] Her position, moreover, calls Brecht ian attention to her status as a woman who "performs" not only within the literal cage at the zoo (and one might think here, too, of the popularity of caged go-go dancers), but also within the metaphorical cage of patriarchal culture.

By eating in public, Sherk makes herself part of a performative display. I began this essay by mentioning that self-consciousness about public eating can be, for women, symptomatic of a larger fear of their own hunger, their own appetites, and ultimately their own bodies. This, of course, is an issue that has frequently been addressed by feminist writers on women, eating, and body image, including Kim Chernin, Susie Orbach, and Susan Bordo (see Chernin 1981 and 1985, Orbach 1978, and Bordo 1993). Not surprisingly, several women performance artists have chosen to address the ways they have been implicated in the cultural obsession with idealized female body images and the subsequent effects on the way they approach food and eating. In Vanalyne Green's *Trick or Drink* (1984), Green used family photographs, children's books, and excerpts from her own diaries to create an autobiographical narrative that explored—in a performance that called for direct audience address and eye contact—her bulimia and weight obsessions as a teenager and its connections to other kinds of addiction in her life (her parents' alcoholism, her own later sexual addictions). The performance—unlike the testimony in, say, a twelve-step program—did not *emphasize* a confessional stance or a movement toward completion and catharsis. Rather, as Sue Ellen Case puts it, *Trick or Drink* was a representation or enactment of Green's "internal growth" (Case 1988, 60).

A more dramatic physical performance of the effect of the aesthetic coding of women's bodies was Eleanor Antin's *Carving*. During the period from July 15 to August 21, 1972, Antin kept herself on a strict diet and had herself photographed, naked, from the same four angles every morning. The photographic series thus depicts Antin's body being "carved" thinner and thinner. The sculptor is, of course, the "hunger artist" Antin herself. Yet it is society's artistic/aesthetic "ideal" of the woman's body that sets the contours of the image that Antin's body-sculpture aims for, but never quite achieves. In other words, by following the diet explicitly for the purpose of the performance/photographs, Antin foregrounds the purely aesthetic outcome of dieting—the sculpting of the body—and as a result provides an almost parodically clinical visual representation of what is "normally" a private, emotional, and psychological cultural obsession. This attitude is clear in Antin's textual commentary on the photographs, throughout which she refers to her body as "the material" and to the period of the dieting as the "carving" of a "work" according to the traditional Greek method of starting with a thick block and removing a layer at a time from all four sides of the block.

She concludes by saying that the sculpture always falls short of the artist's idealized image. She quotes Michelangelo: *non ho l'ottimo artista alcun concetto che el marmo solo non in se circoscrive,* or "not even the greatest sculptor can make anything that isn't already inside the marble" (Antin 1981, 62). In *The Object of Performance,* Henry Sayre provides an interesting commentary:

> Antin's "ideal image" of herself is clearly problematized terrain, tied up, as it is, in dieting, in an image of a woman inspired by the fashion and fitness industries, in a mystique of thinness that, if nothing else, would require Antin to be at least a foot taller than she is . . . What her work underscores is her *difference* from the ideal, even as she subscribes (with tongue in cheek) to its codes. But the real message here is that, before submitting herself to carving, before dieting, Antin is not perceived to be "lifelike." She is a block of matter, awaiting animation by the sculptor's hand. (Sayre 1989, 78)

While I agree with Sayre that Antin's unachieved "ideal image" is "problematized terrain," it seems to me that Sayre himself (in, for example, the comment that Antin would need to be taller) has assumed both the culturally sanctioned physical ideal and, to some degree, Antin's acceptance of it. I would be more inclined to bring Sayre's parenthetical "tongue in cheek" out of the parentheses, to suggest Antin's agency in her position as subject—as the artist—even while she ironically renders herself as an object (i.e., both of sculpture and of the photographs). That is, I would read Antin's performance with, rather than against, its textual commentary. The work's resonance is less in Antin's psychological sense of her shortcomings as artist/sculpture than in her defiant act of making the so-called failure of her piece into the material of the performance itself.

In "Fear of Dining and Dining Conversation" (1981), a piece that its creator, Ellen Zweig, says should ideally be performed in a place where people are sitting at tables and eating (and possibly with dancers who also stop and occasionally peel potatoes), uses the verbal texts of food to confront the complications of women's appetites in a culture that attempts to suppress them. The piece is done with two voices; one of them recites a pastiche of food names, definitions of cooking terms, and calorie counts, while the other voice is a rhythmic prose poem about the fear of eating, punctuated with variations on the title phrase:

> Fear of dining and dining conversation, acts of power and manipulation. She wanted a little cake, something she could carry with her. She could take little bites of the cake, keeping it hidden. A small boy is

eating, meaning to expand. Fear of eating and eating conversation, acts
of power and false termination. (Zweig 1981, 56)

Some of the phrases of the first voice (e.g., "to blend a fragile mixture")
take on wider metaphorical references when heard in counterpoint to the
second voice's narrative of fear and denial ("she begins to mortify herself,
by fasting and immoderate hikes" [Zweig 1981, 57–58]). The second
voice, which seems to be inspired by the material in Kim Chernin's study
on women and food, *The Obsession*, moves into an emphasis on starvation
at the same time that the first voice speaks about Ellen West (a woman
whose self-starvation is discussed by Chernin and others—and whose
name, interestingly, resembles that of Ellen Zweig). The two voices come
together at the end with the words, "No matter what you say./No matter
what you say./There is no solace./There is no consolation" (Zweig 1981,
58; see also the discussion of Ellen West in Chernin 1981, esp. 162–79).
Zweig's piece creates a sense of the ways that food has been inscripted, or
entextualized, upon the bodies of its preparers and consumers. The litany
of recipes and calorie counts, especially when heard in conjunction with
the nightmarish repetitions of food-related compulsions and neuroses,
suggests that the distinction between what one does to food and what the
woman does to herself (or has done to her) has broken down; what is left
are textual fragments (echoed in the emphasis throughout on blanching,
reducing, boiling, chopping) that mark a history of repression and denial,
embodied ultimately in the historical figure of West. At the same time,
perhaps Zweig's preference for having the piece performed in a room
where people are eating together at tables suggests an impulse for breaking through the "fear of dining" by creating a sense of community.

Suzanne Lacy, whose works were mentioned once already in this
chapter in the context of meat-eating, places even greater emphasis on
this notion of the community in her pieces' literal and metaphorical use
of the "potluck." Food, says Lacy in an interview with Linda Montano,
"serves as a bridge between private rituals and social issues" (Montano
1981, 49). In an early group piece for women, for example, Lacy says that
everyone performed their images of food, and an enormous amount of
anger emerged: among others, one participant "crammed food down her
doll's mouth while someone else passed around Valentine chocolate candies filled with glass and nails" (Montano 1981, 49). As a result, the group
"discovered a close connection between food and insanity." Lacy's later
pieces, inspired by Judy Chicago's *Dinner Party*, sought to create healing
ways for expressing women's relationships to food; she began by setting
up a series of potlucks "probably because it's a metaphor for nurturing
each other" (Montano 1981, 49). Lucy Lippard points out that the potluck
allows Lacy to work through a prototypically feminist organizing structure (like that of a quilting party), and it also contains elements of ritual,
as well as providing accessibility to a diverse group of women:

Women who would never come to a meeting because they feel they have "nothing to contribute" will bring food to a potluck. Women traditionally allow the rest of the world to feed off their own bodies and lives, as epitomized by a Tlingit potlach trough (owned by the Denver Museum of Natural History) in the form of a huge, disemboweled female body. Embraced by the healing framework of Lacy's art, women "make sacrifices" only to each other, and for the good of the female community. (Lippard 1988, 74)

Although she does risk some degree of homogenization by attempting to use the "potluck" to bring together women of all ages, races, and classes (Lippard calls this taking them "in symbolic bites"), Lacy also is aware of the immense power inherent in transforming the private rituals of dining into the public space of shared food and the communal "performance" of consumption (Lippard 1988, 74). Even her slightly later "Whisper" pieces (*Whisper, the Waves, the Wind* [1984], *The Crystal Quilt* [1987]), which do not involve food but which still involve women sitting together at tables, draw upon this image of the dinner party. In all of these pieces, though there may of course be additional onlookers, it is crucial that Lacy blurs the boundaries between performers and spectators by having most of those present be participants; as a result, the spectators themselves perform rather than subjecting "othered" actors to their consuming gaze.

The effect of Lacy's "potluck" performance is to nurture her spectators. For Karen Finley, a performance artist who challenges the consuming gaze in radically different ways, the effect is to confront them—to chew the audience up and spit it out. Finley's works test the boundaries between "acceptable" and "unacceptable" female behavior by staging private behavior in the public space of performance (see my discussion of Finley's work in Geis 1993, 160–66). In Finley's pieces, food frequently becomes a device for underscoring the female body's appropriation as object of desire in a consumer culture. If, as Maria Nadotti puts it, the "language of seduction" is "an obligatory instrument in any practice of consumption," then Finley makes use of the ways products like "designer" food take advantage of sexualized forms of capitalist greed and longing (Nadotti 1989, 114). Her works frequently fantasize a scatological sabotaging of this food, using the body to desecrate and decorate that which goes into the body. In *The Family that Never Was*, Finley says:

> Then I see what's in those diary cases. It's that Frudgen Gladge [*sic*], that Haggen-Dazs, that Ben and Cherry Garcia ice cream bullshit that's ruining my culture. That $12.99-a-pint-cream. Then I open up all the cartons of ice cream and I piss in 'em, I jerk off in 'em, I fart in 'em. I go into little kids' butts and take their turds and put it into that chocolate macadamia stuff. I stuff it back into the freezer and go back and stand at the great temple of our culture: the video rental counter. (Finley 1990, 39)

If the female body is an object of consumption, then in Finley's work, the literalizing (through performance) of this image becomes a way of expressing anger toward the patriarchy's efforts to reinforce this status; by claiming, exaggerating, and parodying the extremes of such sexual fantasies, Finley is able to enact a Brechtian/Artaudian confrontation of her audience members' roles as consumers of female flesh. Throughout *Quotes from a Hysterical Female,* for instance, the following passage's deliberate address to "the men" within the narrative mirrors Finley's implicit challenge to the men in the audience of her performance:

> The men are upchucking all over the place, and then it's time for our annual sushi party. Well, I open up a can of tuna and I put it into the folds of my vulva. Then I stand in front of the men, over the men, and then I say to the men, "SUSHI PARTY BOYS! EAT UP!" They are all out of their minds from the pills and the puking and they are chewing me, chewing me. Then they say this isn't like usual tuna, it's kinda juicy and soggy. Sushi, sushi, juicy sushi. And they are eating me up. And I've got my party going. (Finley 1990, 48)

By taking the very material (her pussy) that is supposed to be the source of titillation for her audience (both within the narrative and in the theater), and literalizing and exaggerating its status as consumable object, Finley deprives the spectators of their opportunity to "feed" upon her. As Nadotti says, she issues "an invitation to voyeurism so hyperbolic that it deactivates itself in the very act of its production" (Nadotti 1989, 114).

Food in Finley's work is frequently connected to violation: the combinations of the domestic and the sexual are rendered comic and shocking, but also all the more disturbing, by the ways that Freudian connections between eating and the body—as in the passage cited above—are deconstructed so that the narrator enacts the most primal fantasies of violation and consumption imaginable. In *The Constant State of Desire,* incest taboos are imaged in terms of transgressive eating, especially in the consecutive sequences of "First Sexual Experience, Laundromat," in which the speaker describes his mother, after he has fucked her in the ass, sucked his own cum out of her asshole, and spit it back into her mouth, as saying "Boy, you got lazy ass cum. You can cum on my pancakes anytime," and "Refrigerator," in which the little girl's father puts her in the fridge, "opens up the vegetable bin . . . [and] starts working on my little hole" (Finley 1988, 148).[5] The sequence concludes with the mother arriving home and saying to the daughter, "Whatever happened to the vegetables for the dinner for tonight? You've been playing with your food, girl! I wanted to make your daddy's favorite" (Finley 1988, 148). Vivian Patraka has a helpful reading of the way these incest passages, with their emphasis on the scatological, dramatize Finley's focus on the performance of "damage":

What is embedded in her language and her gestures is the resulting breakdown of distinctions, even among the organs and products of the body, and the confusion of taking in and putting out, the traumatic shock to the directional signals of the girl child body, in its violation by an adult male. The scatological functions partly as protest, expressed in what comes out of the body, to what should never have been taken into it, and partly as a shitty enactment of the violation (of interior space, projected outward by Finley to invade the performative space). What issues forth, thus, in Finley's text is not the semiotic, it is history issuing from a female body. And it is the end, not the beginning, of seduction, desire constant because it is frozen, back in the ice-box of violation. (Patraka 1992, 172)

As the title of Finley's piece (which is her "answer" both to Freud and to Betty Friedan's *The Feminine Mystique*) suggests, the "constant state" of desire is addressed on several levels; sexual desire and the desire to "consume" another being is conflated with the capitalist desire to acquire, to take, to feed off of others—and ultimately, the theater audience's concurrent desire to be titillated implicates them in the very fantasies of transgression, which they have paid to be shocked and disgusted by in Finley's performance itself (as Jeanie Forte points out, this is also what is implicitly appealed to or misleadingly "promised" in the title [Forte 1992, 257]). Finley makes this connection even more explicit in the "chocolate balls" sequence of *The Constant State of Desire*. The narrative of cutting off the testicles of Wall Street traders and making them into chocolate candies to sell in "gourmet chocolate shops" (Finley 1988, 142) creates a simultaneously castrating and scatological image as a parodic comeback to the male audience's desire to consume the female body; in response, Finley imaginatively appropriates and consumes the bodies of her spectators.

While the spoken texts of Finley's works invoke images of food, the visual counterparts body forth the metaphorical connections between eating and sexuality. In *The Constant State of Desire*, Finley at one point smashes uncooked colored Easter eggs in a plastic bag with stuffed animals, and applies the egg mixture to her nude body "using soaked animals as applicators"; at another point, she tosses candies to the audience (Finley 1988, 140). One portion of *We Keep Our Victims Ready* involves Finley smearing melted chocolate on her bare torso; as she explains in an interview with Andrea Juno, the chocolate "ritual" (as she likes to call it), like the "chocolate balls" sequence of *The Constant State of Desire*, allows her to conflate eating, sexuality, and excretion—only the image is even more powerful as it is made visual:

I could use *real* shit, but we know that happens already . . . I use chocolate because it's a visual symbol that involves eating as well as basically being treated like shit . . . so it works on different levels. There are so many occasions where you go into a job or situation and you just have to *eat the shit*—there's no other way out.

Then I stick little candy hearts (symbolizing "love") all over my body—because after we've been treated like shit, then we're loved. And many times that's the only way people *get* love. Then I add the alfalfa sprouts (symbolizing sperm) because in a way it's all a big jack-off—we're all being jerked off . . . we're just something to jerk off onto, after the "love." Finally, I put tinsel on my body, because after going through all that, a woman still gets dressed up for dinner. (Juno 1991, 49)

In Finley's multiple-performer piece *The Theory of Total Blame* (1988), the family is gathered for Thanksgiving dinner; in Shepardian style, a tremendous, sickening quantity of food covers the table and spills from the refrigerator—but remains uneaten. As the mother prepares and serves the food (jello, meatloaf), she also renders it inedible as her children refuse it. Nadotti argues that in this piece "as elsewhere in Finley's work, what is ordinarily considered consumable is . . . transformed into a threatening signifier of reciprocal aggression" (Nadotti 1989, 115). Excessive food is, as Coward suggests, one of the ritual elements of festive eating in its demonstration of "profusion and survival" (Coward 1985, 111). If the food seems to reproduce itself endlessly, though, for Finley this becomes part of its *un*consumability; once again, the exaggeration forces the spectators to reexamine their own literal and metaphorical hungers.

In *Gender Trouble*, Judith Butler suggests that even what we would consider the "interior essence" of the gendered body is in itself a kind of fabrication, as "that very interiority is a function of a decidedly public and social discourse, the public regulation of fantasy through the surface politics of the body" (Butler 1990, 136). The "performance" of eating (in the sense of performance art, though I would argue, again, that any kind of public eating is always, to some degree, a performance), because it is so intimately connected with the gendering of the "eater," is one of the ways that this interiority is expressed through the body politic(s). (And as the next chapter will demonstrate, that body politic is marked by race as well as by gender.) Rosalind Coward's synecdochal image of the mouth for women as a "site of drama" takes Butler's assertion one step further. "When women attempt to lay claim to the pleasures of the mouth," says Coward, "they are often constricted by anxiety about transgressing the appropriate expression of female desire" (Coward 1985, 122). Both Butler and Coward are suggesting that the sites of possible transgressive activity are socially constricted by the rules of public performance; since performance art provides a relatively "safe" area in which to challenge these rules, expressions of appetite and desire can be exaggerated, parodied, resexualized or desexualized, liberated, questioned, and deconstructed. There is always, after all, an audience eager to be fed.

NOTES

1. In a long-running popular entertainment piece called *Tony 'n' Tina's Wedding*, the spectators participated in eating a catered wedding dinner (of Italian food) as part of the simulated ceremony and reception. Just as the piece played at making the spectators into "performers" (as they were invited to participate in the events of the "wedding" and as the actors improvised with them), the actors joined them as "consumers" in the communal act of eating. Thus, although the piece was intended as a parody of the ritual events of weddings, it took on its own ritual qualities in performance.

2. I am inclined to agree with Jeanie Forte's argument that a feminist analysis can include a reading that joins the material body with the body as a cultural construct. The latter, when seen in terms of "the body in representation," provides a way of approaching feminist performance in particular. See Forte 1992, 249.

3. For further discussion, see Jameson 1991. Pierre Bourdieu suggests that the body is a materialization of class taste. According to Bourdieu, not only are certain foods perceived in Western culture as masculine or feminine, but "male" and "female" ways of eating (e.g, gulping vs. nibbling), involving respectively the back and the front of the mouth, can be compared to the ways men and women use their mouths for talking in social situations. See Bourdieu 1984, 190–92.

4. One might think, for instance, about people watching chimps at the zoo: we see them pick their noses, defecate, etc.—all "private" acts that an audience is not, at least as far as other people are concerned, "supposed" to watch. Sherk's piece also reminds me of a tour I once took of the CNN complex in Atlanta; the tour group was given a closed-circuit view of the "off-camera" Headline News anchor in the "cage" of the anchor booth/TV monitor so that an audience watches her scratching herself, yawning, and so forth (a real violation, I would argue, of her privacy).

5. According to Rosalind Coward, "the boy child . . . never loses the possibility of restoring the mother's body as sexual object, and therefore the possibility of regarding sexual gratification as a form of nurturing." She points out, citing Melanie Klein's work on infantile fantasies of devouring the mother, that the language of affection is also very much a language of sadism when it implies the devouring or consuming of the love object" (Coward 1985, 89).

FIVE

The Last Black Man's Fried Chicken

*Soul Food, Memory, and African
American Culinary Writing*

As Michael W. Twitty writes in his recent memoir/study of Southern African American culinary traditions, *The Cooking Gene*, "There is no chef without a homeland" (Twitty 2017, 6). He cautions, though, against those who "take for granted their fast and easy connections to a food narrative that grounds them in a tradition" but who do so in a way that is "blissfully apolitical" (Twitty 2017, 7). Just as the performance artists described in the previous chapter take the body politics of food very seriously (even in the playfulness of their performances), the writers whose works I will discuss here are deeply concerned, even in the midst of demonstrating their creative and culinary prowess, about the connections between a cooking tradition—in this case, "soul food"—and its larger political implications. My focus here is primarily on works by playwright Suzan-Lori Parks and chef/memoirist Jeff Henderson, but I will also invoke the late great playwright/poet Ntozake Shange, who wrote repeatedly about food, in various genres, throughout her career. Parks's play *Death of the Last Black Man in the Whole Entire World* and Henderson's food memoir *Cooked* invoke and question soul food's connection to the African-American past. Parks's play is a choral piece in which a condemned Black man, forced to die over and over, is fed fried chicken by the iconically named Black Woman with Fried Drumstick. Henderson's memoir covers his journey from "cooking" (and dealing) crack cocaine to becoming the first African-American executive chef at the Bellagio in Las Vegas.

Parks, a celebrated contemporary African American playwright (she was the first Black woman to win the Pulitzer Prize in Drama for her

Topdog/Underdog in 2002), returns repeatedly to images of food in her works. In the very early one-act play *Pickling*, the eccentric protagonist "preserves" her memories in pickle jars; in *Venus*, the title character of the Venus Hottentot (based on the real Saartje Baartman) is seduced by chocolates and the play itself includes both a monologue about the history of chocolate and a Glossary of Chocolates. In *Topdog/Underdog*, ill-fated brother Booth and Lincoln dine on takeout shrimp together after payday, and Booth sets forth an elaborate dinner for his girlfriend Grace, who stands him up. In her two takes on Nathaniel Hawthorne's *The Scarlet Letter*, Hester in the first play (*In the Blood*) attempts to feed her starving children by getting them to imagine that their watery soup has everything from pie to diamonds in it, and in the second play (*Fucking A*), branded with a scarlet "A" (for Abortionist) on her chest, Hester's most understanding companion is a Butcher who sings a song about a Meat Man as eligible marriage material. And in Parks's recent work, the Civil War epic *Father Comes Home from the Wars*, the slaves' spoons are among their most precious possessions. Food and hunger, for Parks, are related to power or the lack thereof, and nowhere is this more clearly demonstrated than in *Last Black Man*.

In the mid-1970s, playwright Ntozake Shange broke new ground with her "choreopoem" entitled *for colored girls who have considered suicide/when the rainbow is enuf*. Not only was this the first play by an African American woman since Lorraine Hansberry's *Raisin in the Sun* to achieve (inter)national recognition, but Shange's style broke all of the rules about Western punctuation and grammar; the words in the piece are designed to dance across the page and to reflect the performance of community. Parks has cited Shange as a major influence on her own boundary-breaking style (Geis 2008, 8–9). More than that, in this and in her subsequent works across different genres, Shange pays consistent attention to the multifaceted and international origins of African American food cultures in a way that helps us to see why both Parks and Henderson are also invested in this history. In the Prologue to her study *Black Hunger*, Doris Witt talks about how reading Shange's novel *Sassafrass, Cypress & Indigo*, in which recipes constitute a central aspect of the narrative, was crucial to her reading of African American women's performative texts:

> *Sassafrass, Cypress & Indigo* requires not simply to be read or spoken (or even viewed in a theater); it demands instead that we perform and consume it—that we cook and eat its recipes as an integral part of our experience of the work. Given the well-known history of black women's exploitation as domestic servants . . . the dual symbolic import of Shange's innovation should be evident. She takes on the role not of cook but of cookbook author, a role long denied to African Americans in a country where it was illegal for slaves to learn to read and write. By incorporating the performance of cooking into novelistic art, moreover, Shange insists that the forms of creative expression long attrib-

uted to African American women should be valued as highly as are the forms often reserved for whites and men. (Witt 1999, 11)

As a continuation of her investment in the history of African American cuisine, as well as a means of expressing its significance to her own life without the veil of fiction, Shange in 1998 wrote *if I can Cook/ you KNow God can*. The book is a memoir and travel journal that is also an erudite cultural studies essay and a cookbook of personal recipes; in her Foreword, Vertamae Smart Grosvenor (whose own work will be discussed shortly) talks about how the "heritage [of African American cuisine] has been a confounding, embarrassing, and frightening inheritance for many. Zaki [Shange] travels through it courageously" (Shange 1998, xiii). In the discussion that follows, I will return several times to Shange's memoir as I explore how Parks and Henderson, too, use performative writing techniques to open up our understanding of the layers of African American culinary history.

While Parks's play and Henderson's memoir may appear to have little in common (other than Black authorship), they actually display similarly ironic and ambivalent attitudes toward the eating of soul food as a public means of honoring African-American memory. Parks, who is concerned in all her plays with the process of "re-membering" Black history, shows how attempts to nurture the eponymous Black Man are nearly overridden by the determination of the media and the dominant culture to obliterate him. And Henderson, while professing the power of soul food in his memories of learning "jailhouse cooking," is torn between affirming this legacy and renouncing it in favor of French-style haute cuisine. Ultimately, though, both writers demonstrate the power of a proactive "consumption" of the past.

Before turning to Parks's and Henderson's specific uses of fried chicken (and other soul food) as iconic images in their works, I'd like to provide some context for how and why "soul food" (and fried chicken in particular) has taken on such cultural weight. Jessica B. Harris, in her landmark cookbook *The Welcome Table* and in her important historical survey *High on the Hog*, reminds us of the origins of such food in the era of slavery. She eschews romanticized accounts of slaves smuggling African foods like okra by reminding us that the truth was that the slave traders themselves "needed to feed slaves a diet on which they would survive" (Harris 2012, 30), so they negotiated trades with African locals to obtain inexpensive foods. Not just food itself, but also traditions connected with food, can be connected to the forced migrations from Africa to the United States; as Harris writes, "Recipes, religious celebrations, meals, menus, and more from the African continent were a part of the cultural baggage that was brought across the Atlantic by those who would be enslaved" (Harris 2012, 15).

In an essay collection edited by Anne Bower called *African-American Foodways*, two writers—William C. Whit and Anne Yentsch—talk about how what we now call soul food emerged from African cooking as reinvented by slaves in the American south as they were forced to work with the scraps they were given—the supposedly less desirable parts of the pig, for instance—and as they grew what they could (greens, yams) in the earth. Some foods, like collard greens, were cooked slowly, while others, like fried chicken, were cooked quickly in hot oil as a way to keep them portable and less perishable. As Whit writes, "A basic division (with some overlap) existed during slavery between food that the cook, usually an African American slave, prepared for the white master's family and that she or he prepared for the African American field worker" (Whit 2009, 51). And as Yentsch puts it, "Both prejudice and poverty forced pre- and post-Civil War African Americans to create a cohesive cooking tradition built with limited resources and making do" (Yentsch 2009, 85). What began as a necessity, however, soon became a coveted cuisine, one that made its way into the plantation houses and that sometimes became a (meager) source of income for former slave cooks after emancipation. In the cookbooks first published by the National Council of Negro women in the 1950s, though, as Anne Bower points out in an essay in the same collection, there was a tendency to shy away from direct references to the African roots of some of these foods; moreover, rather than mentioning chitterlings, pigs feet, and other delicacies, the books include a lot of more mainstream recipes for broiled steak, veal, frozen green beans, and so forth (Bower 2009, 159–60).

As Doris Witt discusses in her fascinating history of debates over soul food in the 1960s, the era of the Black Power movement was one in which soul food was caught between the past and the present. In 1962, LeRoi Jones (later Amiri Baraka) published an essay called "Soul Food" in his collection *Home*, lauding the foods such as chitterlings, hog maws, and neckbones that "ofays seldom get to peck" (qtd. in Witt 1999, 82). Citing chicken as an especially fraught object of desire because in slave culture it may have been obtained on the sly, Baraka writes, "People kill chickens all over the world, but chasing them through the dark on somebody else's property would probably insure, once they went in the big bag, that you'd find some really beautiful way to eat them. I mean, after all the risk involved" (qtd. in Witt 1999, 88). As Witt goes on to discuss, though, part of the controversy over soul food came with the rise of the Nation of Islam: since pork was integral to soul food but was seen by Muslims as an unclean and forbidden food, Elijah Muhammad and others condemned its consumption (Witt 1999, 107). Only in the following decade, with the interest in cookbooks by Vertamae Smart-Grosvenor (*Vibration Cooking*) and others that claimed a return to diasporic foodways and a reclaiming of the African-American past, was soul food recuperated as politically correct. William Whit aptly suggests that "soul food demonstrates the manner in which, in the face of unfavorable social conditions, slaves involved themselves collectively in creating a new cuisine that addressed problems of nutritional adequacy and ethnic and racial identity" (Whit 2009, 55). And Harris describes the difficulty of defining exactly what soul food is, saying that it depends on an "ineffable quality" that combines multiple aspects of Black history, from Africa to slavery to Reconstruction to the Harlem Renaissance and after:

> It is a combination of nostalgia for and pride in the food of those who came before. In the manner of the Negro spiritual "How I Got Over," soul food looks back at the past and celebrates a genuine taste palate while offering more than a nod to the history of disenfranchisement of blacks in the United States. In the 1960s, as the history of African Americans began to be rewritten with pride instead of with the shame that had previously accompanied the experience of disenfranchisement and enslavement, soul food was as much an affirmation as a diet. Eating neckbones and chitterlings, turnip greens and fried chicken, became a political statement for many, and African American restaurants that had existed since the early part of the century were increasingly being patronized not only by blacks but also by those in sympathy with the movement. (Harris 2012, 208)

A parallel complex history exists of the "mammy," the Black woman in the kitchen of the Old South who was supposedly the provider and sustainer of the white plantation household. Her presence, retained in popular culture through *Gone with the Wind* and other works, has lasted for more than a century as the mythic and symbolic figure of the Black woman in the kitchen. M.M. Manring's *Slave in a Box*, a compelling narrative of the endurance in American culture of the Aunt Jemima figure (who still exists, though in a slightly different form, on pancake mixes that bear her name), remarks, "If the mammy had not possessed such a strong hold on American literary and historical imagination, Aunt Jemima never would have become a powerful advertising trademark" (Manring 1998, 20). Manring's explanation of why the much-beloved mammy character sustained the romanticization of slavery is worth quoting in full because it helps us to understand why writers like Parks, partly in response to Margaret Mitchell, William Faulkner, and many other American novelists, would attempt to resurrect and re-member her. Manring says:

> The mammy was a key ingredient in the Old South fable because of her role among its happy, devoted slaves. As the servant and biological opposite of the delicate, pure, ultrafeminine southern woman of the Old South, the large, strong, sexless mammy provided a needed contrast. As "the foremost Big House slave," she not only complemented white womanhood but served as the home's domestic manager. She was more than a servant of white folks; the mammy of the Old South mythology was a collaborator in their society, a reassuring figure who,

despite her breeding, comforted her white betters, offered advice, kept black males in line, and put hot food on the table. However the image of the mammy might not have squared with reality, it soothed white guilt over slavery and uplifted white womanhood through sheer contrast and by keeping white women out of the kitchen. She saved them from work but also from worry and seemingly cleared up tensions between white men and white women, between masters and servants, by clarifying sexual and work roles as well as racial lines. (Manring 1998, 22–23)

In *Building Houses Out of Chicken Legs: Black Women, Food, & Power*, Psyche Williams-Forson bases an entire—and utterly gripping—study on the history of fried chicken as an iconic African-American food, concentrating on particular on the way that the association with fried chicken fostered stereotypes of Black women, in the early twentieth century, as mammies. In the advertising, the postcards, and even the fiction of this period, she demonstrates, myriad images "of the mammified black woman [preparing] . . . fried chicken . . . attempted to reinforce multiple stereotypes of black women" (Williams-Forson 2006, 86). However, when Williams-Forson interviewed a group of contemporary female African-American church members at the time she was working on this study, the insistence on the importance of fried chicken—especially for a journey—was still utterly prevalent. She argues:

By utilizing and identifying symbols (like foods) that are commonly affiliated with African-American cultural heritage, black people refuse to allow the wider American culture to dictate what represents acceptable notions of their expressive culture. (Williams-Forson 2006, 128)

She goes on to use examples from her own experience to argue that "chicken serves as an overarching symbol of identity in the travel narratives of some African-Americans" (Williams-Forson 2006, 128). And in fact, we see fried chicken being used this way in the repeated journeys to and from the world of the dead in Suzan-Lori Parks' *Death of the Last Black Man in the Whole Entire World*.

When the Black Man with Watermelon in Parks's play returns from the dead, the first thing that the Black Woman with Fried Drumstick does is to try to comfort him with food: "Cold compress then some hen" (Parks 1995a, 105). As she tells him the story of his demise, he looks wonderingly at the watermelon he is holding and disavows any connection to it: "Saint mines . . . This does not belong tuh me. Somebody planted this on me. On me in my hands" (Parks 1995a, 105). The way the Black Man is attached to the watermelon—it is even part of his character's name—speaks to the complicated history of watermelon in African American culture as both a cherished food item and a hated stereotype (the subject of an endless number of racist caricatures and knickknacks). He says that it isn't his—he wonders who gave birth to it—and yet he can't let go of it. Jessica Harris talks about watermelon and its difficult role:

> Watermelons arrived in the continental United States fairly early on in the seventeenth century and were taken to heart and stomach rapidly as new cultivars were developed that were more suitable to the cooler weather. As with okra, watermelon has been indelibly connected to African Americans. Indeed some of the most virulently racist images of African Americans produced in the post-Civil War era involve African Americans and the fruit. Watermelon became so stereotypically African American that black comedian Godfrey Cambridge in the 1960s developed a comedy routine about the travails of an upwardly mobile black man trying to bring home a watermelon without being seen by the neighbors in his upscale white community. He declared that he couldn't wait until a square watermelon was developed that would defy detection . . . National attitudes toward watermelon have changed, but the fruit and its stereotyped history still remain a hot-button issue for many. (Harris 2012, 17–18)

Bower's discussion of mid-twentieth century African American cook-books also plays out this ambivalent relationship with what she calls "that food so stereotyped as part of black culture that to this day some African Americans will not eat it in public" (Bower 2009, 160). In the cookbook, Bower points out, watermelon appears in the form of recipes for pickled watermelon rind and for watermelon sherbet (eaten in a gen-teel fashion with a spoon)—but its appeal as a fruit eaten raw is never mentioned. In her memoir, Shange recalls her childhood frustration at loving watermelon but being given warnings about when to consume it:

> The watermelon is an integral part of our actual life as much as it is a feature of our stereotypical lives in the movies, posters, racial jokes, toys, and early American portraits of the "happy darky." We could just as easily been eatin' watermelon in D.W. Griffiths' *Birth of a Nation* as chicken legs. The implications are the same . . . I remember being in-structed not to order watermelon in restaurants or to eat watermelon in any public places because it makes white people think poorly of us. They already did that, so I don't see what the watermelon was going to precipitate . . . In my rebelliousness as a child, I got so angry about the status of the watermelon, I tried to grow some in the flower box on our front porch in Missouri. My harvest was minimal to say the least. (Shange 1998, 45)

Witt, too, alludes to the way that watermelon was perceived in the Civil Rights and Black Power era as "a trenchant symbol of the oft-precarious status of U.S. racial and gender identities" (Witt 1999, 127), citing Melvin Van Peebles's 1970 film *Watermelon Man* as an example of a work of art that played with this trope. She also quotes activist Dick Gregory as saying in his second autobiography that he "often used a watermelon as a sort of personal symbol and a private joke. For years, white folks have enjoyed poking fun at Black folks' fondness for watermelon. I reversed the process and made the watermelon a symbol of pride in Blackness" (qtd. in Witt 1999, 47). Parks's Black Man with Watermelon, like Gregory and like contemporary poet Terrance Hayes whose "Sonnet" repeats the line, "We sliced the watermelon into smiles" (Hayes 2002, 13), allows us to contemplate the watermelon, then, as both loved and hated symbol. "This thing dont look like me!" the Black Man says (Parks 1995a, 106), and wonders, "Was we green and stripedly when we first comed out?" (Parks 1995a, 107).

The Black Woman in this play is a powerful figure, in history as in the way she is represented here; as Nicole Hodges Persley puts it, "Parks positions Black Woman with Fried Drumstick as the narrator of [the] story, a wife who is charged with supporting her husband and with being a leader in the community that surrounds her" (Persley 2010, 69). She keeps offering the Black Man food and he refuses repeatedly, saying, "Last meal I had was my last-mans-meal" (Parks 1995a, 106). There is an uncomfortable equation made between his condemned body and his condemned meal as the Black Woman describes how they "woulda fried" him (like the chicken) "right here on thuh front porch but we dont got enough electric" (Parks 1995a, 107); instead, when the electric chair is placed on the town square, "Folks come tuh watch with picnic baskets" (Parks 1995a, 107). As with lynchings in the Old South, his death becomes a spectator sport.

Throughout the play, he dies again and again; at one point, when he has trouble breathing and the Black Woman loosens his collar, he has been lynched and has a noose tied to a tree branch still hanging from his neck. Later, the Black Man is willing to eat when he says that he is able to remember "what I like. I remember what my likes tuh eat when I be in thuh eatin mode" (Parks 1995a, 125). Having an identity, or trying to, is about being able to make choices, and so he attempts to figure out who he is by remembering what he likes to eat:

> Choice between peas and corns—my feets—. Choice: peas. Choice between peas and greens choice: greens. Choice between greens and potatoes choice: potatoes. Yams. Boiled or mashed choice: mashed. Aaah. Mmm. My likenesses. (Parks 1995a, 125)

And so she is able to feed him, but the image of "stuffin" or being "stuffed" (Parks 1995a, 127) is conflated with the image of the taxidermied body; thus, it is again his "last-mans-meal." The Black Woman with Fried Drumstick tries to re-member the Black Man with Watermelon— that is, to put him back together. She says, "he have uh head he been keepin under thuh Tee V. On his bottom pantry shelf. He have uh head that hurts. Dont fit right" (Parks 1995a, 102). Her attempt to restore him includes chopping the heads off of "[e]very hen on the block" (Parks 1995a, 106). She tells of the neighbors turning on her as a result, also claiming that the hens "eat their own," or at least she "[s]aw it on thuh Tee V" (Parks 1995a, 109), but the Black Man, disconnected from himself, simply responds, "Aint that nice" (Parks 1995a, 109). And when we do hear the Voice on Thuh Tee V, it suggests the media's role not in record-ing history but in distorting it: "News of Majors [the last black man's] death sparked controlled displays of jubilation in all corners of the world" (Parks 1995a, 110). The play mourns the loss of a world that used to be "*roun*": "they put uh /d/ on thuh end of roun makin roun*d*. Thusly they set in motion thuh end" (Parks 1995a, 102). In other words, the dominant powers control not just the recording of history but the lan-guage with which history is told. Shange's memoir echoes this emphasis on how and when choices of resistance are possible in the face of oppres-sion; she asks, "When we are illicit, what can we keep down, what do we offer the spirits, the trickster, *el coyote*, who led us from bondage to a liberty so tenuous we sometimes hide for years our right to be?" (Shange 1998, 6). She goes on to give an example of how, given that many of the so-called founding fathers were slaveholders, Frederick Douglass and other abolitionists felt reluctant to celebrate it, choosing instead to honor the New Year: "And so, black-eyed peas and rice or 'Hoppin John,' even collard greens and pigs' feet, are not so much arbitrary predilections of the 'nigra' as they are symbolic defiance; we shall celebrate ourselves on a day of our choosing in honor of those events and souls who are an honor to us" (Shange 1998, 6–7).

The Black Man with Watermelon and the Black Woman with Fried Drumstick are not the only food figures in Parks's play; others include Yes and Greens Black-Eyed Peas Cornbread, Lots of Grease and Lots of Pork, and even Ham (with a pun on the Biblical Hamm). Collard greens have a lengthy history as an integral part of the soul food tradition; originally part of this cuisine because they could be foraged and were not considered desirable enough for the white plantation table, they became a much-loved component of the African American southern table. Shange's unconventionally phrased recipe for collard greens (which she calls "Collard Greens to Bring You Money") in her memoir evokes the southern past when she mentions that "Some folks like their greens chopped just so, like the rows of a field" (Shange 1998, 10). In her signifi-cant 1970 book *Vibration Cooking*, Vertamae Smart Grosvenor tells several anecdotes about greens, one of which involves having a white woman in the supermarket ask her what she is going to do with them. Since Gros-venor was having a particularly bad day, rather than responding that what she had in mind was to cook them up as a source of comfort food, she pretends that she is going to use them for a salad with Italian dress-ing; another black woman who overhears her "looked at me as if I had discredited the race" (qtd. in Witt 1999, 12). She also points out that collard greens are part of other culinary traditions, saying that they were considered a delicacy in the days of the Roman Empire and that "Soul food is more than chitlins and collard greens, ham hocks and black-eyed peas. Soul food is about a people who have a lot of heart and soul" (qtd. in Witt 1999, 159–80). For Parks, soul food is irretrievably a part of the African-American past, so much so that it is "embodied" on stage through these more-than-human characters, stage figures with soul food names. As Yvette Louis points out in her valuable discussion of the Black female body in this play (and as I have cited in my earlier book's consideration of it), "Parks uses food as a powerful metaphoric tool for restoring what has been ruptured on the physical, social, cultural, and linguistic levels. She maximizes food . . . as a vigorous element in re-membering the black body" (Louis 2001, 160).

The name of the character Lots of Grease and Lots of Pork alludes to the prevalence of pork in soul food, namely, again, through pigs' feet, chitterlings, and other items that were devised out of necessity (the parts that the white plantation families didn't want) but that became coveted delicacies. Whit points out that cooking these parts of the pig also fulfills the African dictum using all of a plant or animal. He explains, "They approached it with a traditional African and preindustrial cultural tradition, using the entire food entity. Stomachs, ears, feet, intestines, brains (primarily in head cheese), ribs, back fat, and hocks all assumed prominent roles in what came to be called soul food" (Whit 2009, 48). As Witt says, the place of pork in a soul food diet was called into question with the rise of Islamic Black communities during the Civil Rights era (Witt 1999, 102–25). In Parks's play, Lots of Grease seems to be one of the narrator figures, a keeper and relayer of historical information. (S)he is complemented by the presence of the figure of Ham, whose name suggests not only the Biblical Hamm, as mentioned earlier—as well as Hamlet, or a "ham actor," in his histrionic vaudevillian monologue that provides one of the showstopping moments of the play—but also, of course, the food. Ham hocks might appear regularly in soul food, and are often used to give a depth of flavor to collard greens. As Henry Louis Gates Jr. recalls in his memoir *Colored People*, "If there is a key to unlocking the culinary secrets of the Coleman family, it is that a slab of fatback or a cupful of bacon drippings or a couple of ham hocks and a long simmering time are absolutely essential to a well-cooked vegetable. Cook it till it's *done*, Mama would say" (Gates 2015, 159). But an actual ham might be considered a special treat for a holiday, a coveted reward or an emblem of something that has been promised but not yet delivered: "he gonna give me my ham!" says the character of Hambone repeatedly in August Wilson's 1992 play *Two Trains Running*—but waiting for one's ham is like waiting for Godot (and Beckett [whom Parks has cited as an influence], in another play, also gives the name of Hamm to one of his characters).

Ham's monologue is a mock family tree that details, in old-school minstrelsy style, a kind of genealogy of slavery. He begins with "Ham's Begotten Tree" and a narrative in which "She goned begotten One who in turn begotten Ours" (Parks 1995a, 121) and, with jokes that might remind audience members of the famous "Who's on first" Abbott and Costello routine, he playfully accelerates the speech into a series of such plays on names, with "Themuhns married outside thuh tribe joinin herself with uh man they called WhoDat," and so forth (Parks 1995a, 122). Lots of Grease and Lots of Pork adds, "This list goes oninon"; others add, "Shame on his family"; Old Man River Jordan makes reference to the Biblical story of Ham and Noah; and all of the characters reciting a version of the slave-era Juba chant, "HAM BONE HAM BONE WHERE YOU BEEN ROUN THUH WORLD N BACK A-GAIN" (Parks 1995a, 122–23). Shange calls the Juba "a dance of courtin' known in slave quarters of North America and the Caribbean" (Shange 1998, 41), but it is also a group performance, an act of community and resistance. Just as the Juba was a means of signifying—of using coded language to express more than the surface meaning, a practice going back to African ritual that continues to today and that interests Parks greatly—Ham's speech is also an act of signify-ing. When he resumes his monologue, it is punctuated with footnote numbers (a favorite Parks device) that in this case have no actual foot-notes, and so they look both like a mockup of Biblical scholarship and like mathematical exponents—and with cries of "SOLD!" (Parks 1995a, 124) which depict the way that the auction block of slavery cut African American legacies and family ties (see Geis 2008, 64–65).

The play's "historical" figures, Before Columbus and Queen-then-Pharaoh Hatshepsut, remind us of the danger of forgetting the past. But it is Yes and Greens Black-Eyed Peas Cornbread who says repeatedly: "You will write it down because if you dont write it down then we will come along and tell the future that we did not exist. You will write it down and you will carve it out of a rock" (Parks 1995a, 130–31). As I have discussed elsewhere, in the original production of the play directed by Liz Di-amond, Yes and Greens was portrayed as an "illiterate slave girl" so that the "least enfranchised figure in the play" is the one who repeats these highly significant lines ("Remarks on Parks 2" 2006, 6; Geis 2008, 62). And in the 2006 Cutting Ball Theatre production of the play directed by Rob Melrose, Yes and Greens was again the repository of memory, only this time imaged as an elderly Black church lady in a rocking chair (Geis 2008, 62). In a strangely literal way, then, the soul food is the keeper of memory, the speaker of wisdom, the retainer of the future.

Like Parks's, Jeff Henderson's work engages in questions of the connec-tion between soul food and issues of an African-American identity as created through the past and through memory. While Parks uses the public medium of dramatic performance, Henderson's vehicle is the equally public and performative mode of cooking—and in this case, also, the confessional story or testimonial. *Cooked* is a remarkable memoir about the transition that author Jeff Henderson makes from drug dealer to executive chef; TV watchers may also remember his reality show *The Chef Jeff Project* that followed *Cooked*, in which he attempted to change the lives of young adults like himself by getting them off of the streets and into his version of a culinary boot camp. In 2011, he also edited the *America I AM: Pass It Down Cookbook*, which was published as part of Tavis Smiley's "American I AM: The African American Imprint" touring museum exhibit celebrating African American culture. His Preface begins with his memory of an interview with Maya Angelou a few years earlier in which they talked about their grandparents cooking soul food. Henderson's nostalgic description of his grandfather's cooking here is quite vivid, and yet it omits the more complicated story of his past that we learn by reading his memoir—as well as the path that he had to take to re-embrace soul food in the first place.

Henderson is quite frank in the early portions of *Cooked* about always feeling hungry, and about learning to steal from watching his grandfather take coins from the laundromats where he worked:

> If I was hungry, I'd take money to buy food. And, like I've said, I was hungry all the time. We always had food at Moms's apartment, whether it was government surplus canned fruit, cheese, or peanut butter and jelly. (I hated the government jelly because it came in a can and you couldn't close it once you opened it.) And there were always leftovers that my grandmother would send home with us, so it's not like Moms didn't feed my sister and me. But we craved junk food. We wanted Church's chicken, Jack in the Box, McDonald's, all the stuff we didn't have money for. (Henderson 2007, 15)

We see an immediate connection here between food and need, one that plays itself out throughout the entire memoir. As a teenager, Henderson is drawn increasingly into the world of petty crime, and eventually— through T-Row, his first of many mentors in the book—gets involved in selling drugs and eventually in the world of crack cocaine. One of the painful ironies of the text is that we see through Henderson's careful descriptions of how he "cooked" the crack the talent that, so misused here, only later transforms into his skill as a chef. He explains that since the major L.A. dealers were selling the "recipe" for making crack cocaine for twenty-five or thirty thousand dollars, he knew he was "ready to go get in the kitchen and do it myself" (Henderson 2007, 57). Even his characterization of the kind of business acumen that he had to possess is not without some kind of awareness that he later will use these same kinds of skills when he enters the culinary world: he learns from T-Row that as a dealer, one had to "be a critical thinker to be truly successful. You had to have the qualities of a salesman, you had to be a manipulator and a chameleon to deal with a diverse clientele. You had to be able to convince people to buy your product" (Henderson 2007, 31).

When he receives a lengthy prison sentence, Henderson's life starts to change. He is always hungry in prison, and his initial descriptions of how much he savored the meals that he and his fellow inmates would put together from the visiting room vending machines are particularly poignant; he says "eating food from those machines was like going to a restaurant" (Henderson 2007, 111). Although it marks a significant change in his interest in self-education when he feels drawn to the various Black Muslim political groups in jail, he refuses to convert because that would mean giving up pork. He includes a detailed list of the snack foods that he buys from the prison commissary and remarks that when he and his fellow inmates would pool their ingredients to make nachos, he was always asked to assemble them "since I had a knack for it" (Henderson 2007, 150). The most life-changing event happens when he joins the kitchen crew. Although he starts reluctantly as a pot washer, he soon realizes that the prison cooking detail allows access to plenty of extra food—for again, he is always hungry. There is a clear connection between his attraction to the food in the prison bakery, and his unsatisfied childhood longings:

> Of all the places in the kitchen, the bakery is what really got my attention: the sweet smells, the sugary crusts on all the pies, the cloverleaf dinner rolls with butter seeping out of the creases. I'd always loved sweets. Growing up, we never had a cookie jar in my mom's kitchen. (Henderson 2007, 136)

As a result of trying to learn the ins and outs of the prison kitchen, he meets his first cooking mentor, Big Roy, who was "the shot caller in the main kitchen" (Henderson 2007, 140). What impresses Henderson is that Big Roy understands the connection between food and love:

> His food always reminded me of the flavors of my childhood, and being in my grandmother's kitchen. Big Roy put love into every dish . . . [and he] truly understood the importance of food to an incarcerated man. He gave us his heart and soul in the kitchen and knew that we loved the southern touches in his food. (Henderson 2007, 141)

In fact, it's only when the inmates are preparing a special soul food meal to celebrate Juneteenth that Henderson finally has his chance to jump in and help with the real cooking process: "With no real experience, I grabbed one of the large paddles and began stirring the collard greens that were in a really big kettle" (Henderson 2007, 143). He finally gets noticed by Big Roy and begins volunteering for more and more extra kitchen duty. There is another side, though, to what Henderson learns at this stage. Big Roy is also quite the operator: he has an entire business on the down-low selling extra chicken to the inmates. So it is from Big Roy that Henderson witnesses some of the same kind of hustling that went on in the drug-dealing business, but with food rather than crack as the merchandise.

When Henderson is transferred to a lower-security prison and joins the inmate kitchen crew at Nellis, he meets the chief cook, Friendly Womack, who proves to be Henderson's second significant cooking mentor. Friendly teaches him to make biscuits, pancakes, salad dressings, and other comfort foods that the inmates yearn for. Strikingly, the only recipe Henderson gives us in the entire memoir is for Friendly's Buttermilk Fried Chicken. He says that while fried chicken had been his favorite food for all of his life, he had never known how to prepare it himself until Friendly gave him the recipe, at which point he thought he was "the man" (Henderson 2007, 163). He even persuades Friendly to participate in a successful side hustle of frying extra chicken and smuggling it out of the jailhouse kitchen to sell, adding that even though he was imitating what he had seen Big Roy do, he ensured that "the brothers" received their chicken first and that the white guys got a different batch, as they preferred, of baked chicken (Henderson 2007, 165). When Friendly is released, Henderson finally gets to be the head of the kitchen and to assemble his own crew.

Yet when Henderson himself finally gets out of prison, he is dissuaded of the value of this fried chicken. Like Marcus Samuelsson, whose work I will discuss in chapter 8 of this book, Henderson is well aware of the lack of Black chefs in the world of fine dining. Jessica Harris speculates about the reasons for this lack:

> The question of why so few African American chefs was much debated. Many recognized that the role of chef offered little inducement to those who had been enslaved for centuries, then traditionally relegated to lower-level service roles receiving low pay and no glory. Those who could afford the often-expensive tuitions at culinary schools discovered upon graduation that despite their abilities, they were often ghettoized, and the soul food debate still raged. (Harris 2012, 239)

One of these prominent chefs, Sterling Burpee, later proves to be an important mentor for Henderson. Of even greater impact is that his first professional chef mentor is Robert Gadsby, a Black British chef whose perfectionism and drive have a huge influence, but who also repeatedly advises Henderson not to define himself by his racial identity. Gadsby says:

> Jeff, in this business, it's not about the brothers. It's not about the Latinos or the whites. It's all about talent, it's all about passion. Get out of the brother business . . . And forget about soul food. No one cares about soul food. It's simply one of the most disrespected cuisines in the world. You have to learn progressive American cuisine. That's what I do, and that's what you will learn from me. (Henderson 2007, 189)

When Gadsby catches Henderson using the deep-fryer to prepare fried chicken, he again admonishes him for being interested in soul food: "how many times do I have to tell you that you have to break yourself away from that soul food anyway, Jeff?" (Henderson 2007, 194). Gadsby's rejection of soul food is no doubt due in part to the fact that he is British rather than African-American, but Henderson does little at this point to question his mentor's advice. Although he comments, "You'd think he was a white guy in blackface" (Henderson 2007, 195), he suggests that Gadsby just wanted the recognition of his peers, who happened to be white chefs; in a sidenote, though, Henderson adds that although he, too, wants the respect of his peers, those peers also include his own community. And it's striking that he says he celebrated his first year out of prison by eating at a Los Angeles soul food restaurant.

At this point, he immerses himself in the fine art of architectural plating design, seared foie gras, and *amuses-bouches*. The very detailed descriptions that he uses to show his process of preparing dishes such as a black beluga lentil soup—which he makes as a test for a job at the Ritz Carlton—shows both his loving attention to detail and concern for his craft, and his sometimes-acute performance anxiety. In fact, the narrative strategy that opens the book involves the story of the meal that he prepares in Las Vegas as a tryout for his position at Caesar's Palace; he wants the reader to be immersed in his fine-dining success story before the memoir turns to his misspent youth. Just as Frederick Douglass in his celebrated autobiography says that he educated himself as a writer by complimenting the white youths he encountered on their writing skills, Henderson says that he learned how to prepare some dishes by approaching and flattering chefs who had received formal Culinary Institute of American training. He's not unaware of the connection between the way he and his friend T-Row used to steal cars, and the way he sees fellow chefs lifting recipes from various sources: "I was learning that no top chef is superhuman. I saw them digging through books, poring over magazines, and stealing other people's creations. They were jackers just like T-Row and me. The only difference was the product" (Henderson 2007, 227).

He is also very frank, though, about his co-workers' attempts to sabotage him during this period, by doing things like switching out the salt he is supposed to put on the lamb for sugar, or drawing racist caricatures of him. Many potential employers won't even talk to him because of his prison record. He suffers several crises of confidence, such as when, in an interview, he can't remember the names of all of the classic sauces. And although he longs to be able to show his skill at cooking soul food, he's terrified of including it when he does various tryouts for high-level positions: at an audition for Table One, for instance, he says that since the restaurant had a lot of powerful African American customers, he was tempted to prepare "something southern, something that played on the flavors that most blacks grew up loving, but I was too afraid of being rejected to make the move" (Henderson 2007, 229).

It is only when Henderson gets the job of chef de cuisine at the Palladian Buffet in Caesar's Palace that he has the courage—as part of his renovation of the buffet—to set out some entrees from his prison years, including Friendly's Buttermilk Fried Chicken. Only with the past behind him and with his acquired confidence in haute cuisine does Henderson feel comfortable embracing the food of his past.

In both Parks's play and Henderson's memoir, the protagonist is an African American male who faces metaphorical and literal death, abandonment, imprisonment, and suffocation. The struggle is an ongoing one—Parks's hero dies again and again, and even at the peak of his profession, Henderson tells of finding racist caricatures of himself left by fellow employees who resent his ascendance. Both of these characters battle their own hunger: while Parks's Black Man with Watermelon insists that he is not hungry but ends up "stuffed" with chicken by the Black Woman with Fried Drumstick, Henderson says that his childhood hunger was what drove him to steal in the first place, and the first thing he stole was food. Soul food manifests itself in both works as a strong marker of past legacies, but it is also a contested means of claiming a connection to one's history. By making this claim and letting it be part of the ongoing performance of the present, though—both Parks and Henderson seem to say—the potential exists for a re-membered, re-embodied subject.

SIX

Cooking Up a Storm

Recent Food Memoirs and the Angry Daughter

I turn now from soul food to the women's food memoir, which has become an astonishingly popular genre since the beginning of the 2000s, and specifically to the vexed mother/daughter relationships that get played out with striking frequency in these works. When I began reading through the stack of food memoirs by women that have been published in the past decade or so, what surprised me most was that while many of these writers did indeed grow up with the "Betty Crocker" style of mother that one might expect daughters raised during the late Baby Boomer/ early Gen X generations to have, the relationships with these mothers are far from idealized. Mother was not the source of wisdom in the kitchen; Mother was often cooking for the sake of guests rather than her own children; or Mother was preoccupied with other things and relied on opening cans and defrosting frozen dinners. Or she may have been absent altogether. More than that, though, I was struck by the amount of ambivalence and anger that these foodie daughters seemed to feel toward their mothers. Barbara Johnson points out that "[t]he cultural construction of ideal motherhood suggests that, when asked for a topic involving violence, the chances are very great that motherhood is one of the *last* things people will think of" (Johnson 2003, 77). This "violence" may be emotional, or self-directed; its manifestations can be subtle or deflected.

As Kim Chernin has shown us so powerfully in *The Hungry Self* (and other books), the extreme form in which the daughter enacts her guilt at having caused the mother's sacrifices can sometimes be eating disorders. She writes, "The child who lives through and loves with the mouth is already constructing that hunger knot in which identity, the beginnings of the mother-separation struggle, love, rage, food, and the female body are entangled" (Chernin 1985, 99). It would seem that this is an inward-turning, a self-punishment, which results from the feeling of helplessness over the act of separating from the mother after infancy. Throughout her psychoanalytic study *The Reproduction of Mothering*, Nancy Chodorow talks about how daughters move from identification with the mother to ambivalence to differentiation: "A girl identifies with and is expected to identify with her mother in order to attain her adult feminine identification and learn her adult gender role. At the same time she must be sufficiently differentiated to grow up and experience herself as a separate individual" (Chodorow 1978, 177). The pattern begins, according to Chodorow, with the mother's ambivalence: "They desire both to keep daughters close and to push them into adulthood. This ambivalence in turn creates more anxiety in their daughters and provokes attempts by these daughters to break away" (Chodorow 1978, 135). It is finally the turn away from the mother that "represents independence and individuation, progress, activity, and participation in the real world" (Chodorow 1978, 82). Or as Kelly Oliver puts it in her discussion of Julia Kristeva's work on motherhood, "[t]he mother is made abject to facilitate the separation from her" (Oliver 1992, 71). María Lugones has a powerful description of what it felt like to begin to sense this separation:

> I was disturbed by my not wanting to be what she was. I had a sense of not being quite integrated, my self was missing because I could not identify with her, I could not see myself in her, I could not welcome her world. I saw myself as separate from her, a different sort of being, not quite of the same species. This separation, this lack of love, I saw, and I think that I saw correctly as a lack in myself (not a fault, but a lack). I also see that if this was a lack of love, love cannot be what I was taught. Love has to be rethought, made anew. (Lugones 1992, 88)

The food memoirists I am discussing, while food becomes a preoccupation and a not-always-healthy obsession in their lives, take pleasure in eating and relish their cooking skills, sometimes using them as a way to rebel against the mother's cooking rituals or to gain the mother's attention. Repeatedly in these memoirs, to a surprising degree, we realize that the authors' interest in cooking is often an angry form of communication with their mothers. For some of them, the subsequent act of becoming mothers or surrogate mothers themselves raises questions of their own guilt and ambivalence about food and maternity, sometimes forcing them to see their earlier relationships with their own mothers in a new light. Kristeva comments, "By giving birth, the woman enters into contact with her mother; she becomes, she is her own mother; they are the same continuity differentiating itself" (Kristeva 1980, 239).

It's also worth pointing out that some of the antagonism that these daughters feel toward their mothers is a generational one: most of the mothers in these memoirs were housewives in the era in which there was no expectation that they would work outside of the home. As Laura Shapiro discusses in *Perfection Salad: Women and Cooking at the Turn of the Century*, the advent of household equipment like electric irons, vacuum cleaners, washing machines, and refrigerators in the post-Depression era meant that even though it "still took much of a woman's time to keep house . . . the hard labor aspects of the work had lightened" (Shapiro 2009, 210). After World War II, the pressure of what Shapiro calls a "wholly compliant femininity" (Shapiro 2009, 214)—having the house clean and dinner ready for one's husband when he comes home from work—was tremendous. What we frequently see in these memoirs are mothers who take their own frustrations at being limited to domestic chores out on their daughters, and daughters who on some level pity their mothers' loss of joy but also resent the extent to which they have certain standards of achievement or performance imposed upon them.

In the discussion that follows, I want to highlight these ideas about maternal separation and continuity, food, and ambivalent mother-daughter relationships by exploring works by eight of these memoirists: Ayun Halliday, Julie Powell, Kim Sunée, Laura Schenone, Kate Moses, Gabrielle Hamilton, Diana Abu-Jaber, and Ruth Reichl.

Ayun Halliday's comical and engaging 2006 food memoir, *Dirty Sugar Cookies*, is about a childhood in Indiana that involved both loving and hating food. Halliday grew up daunted by her mother's cooking skills: "My mother, who as a bride had worked her way through Julia Child's *Mastering the Art of French Cooking* dish by dish, was more of a gourmet and thus more of a problem for a child whose sense of culinary adventure was as pinched as mine" (Halliday 2006, 3). She adds, "I've blotted out the specifics of the dishes she labored over for hours, they were so traumatic" (Halliday 2006, 3–4). Although she claims to have taken pride in her family's "grandly appointed formal dining room" (Halliday 2006, 4), she feels the pressure of her mother having abandoned a journalism career in order to raise her and the sense in which this mother now "had all the time in the world to reduce sauces and braise shallots" (Halliday 2006, 4). Apparently Halliday's mother was even profiled at one point in the *Indianapolis Star*'s "Seasoning and Savoring" column in May 1970. Since Halliday was an only child, with "no older siblings to spirit me off to the local pizza parlor, and no younger siblings to exhaust the chef into cracking open a can of SpaghettiOs," she felt instead that she was "held prisoner" to her mother's ambitious culinary creations (Halliday 2006, 4). But Halliday also credits her mother, who adopted the concept of the "courtesy bite" from Halliday's school lunchroom, for transforming her appreciation for new and different food when the two of them went to a Greek café and tried spanokopita: it was "something I wanted to keep on my tongue forever" (Halliday 2006, 65).

Throughout the memoir, Halliday chronicles the paradoxical relationship she developed with food as the result of being both a picky eater and, eventually, an enthusiastic one. In the later parts, beginning with her experience of coming down with deli-induced listeria while pregnant, we can see her facing her own pressures as a mother who must do things like participate in her daughter's kindergarten cookie baking extravaganza. Again, she is haunted by her mother's perfectionism and describes the way her mother insisted upon replicating authentic colonial American recipes: "While other friends were having themselves a gay old time, glopping fluorescent icing and all manner of wang-dang-doodles onto tacky Santas and reindeer, I was carrying out Mistress Betsy's fanatical bidding as sheet after sheet of the molasses-flavored fuckers emerged from the oven" (Halliday 2006, 178). Her own daughter's pickiness, it seems to Halliday, is almost a fated revenge for the battles her mother went through with her. At the end, her discovery of her grandmother's old recipe box brings Halliday and her mother together in an emotional moment, as they discover that the recipes contained therein are not so much dishes to be treasured as social relics that were traded among friends.

In a sense, then, *Dirty Sugar Cookies* is a story in which the mother both creates food as a site of trauma, and becomes a representation of a certain kind of unattainable, idealized feminine domesticity. The daughter simultaneously resists becoming the mother by resisting the mother's culinary visions, yet becomes the mother—becomes a mother—and locates a certain empathy at the heart of all of this resistance. It is striking that the actual recipes throughout the memoir—for the title "dirty sugar cookies" and the like—are phrased as irreverently as possible; the quiche recipe, for example, ends, "if you don't give a raccoon's ass for presentation, dig in!" (Halliday 2006, 51). The style of the recipes is clearly a kind of anti-Julia Child voice, one that the mother would find truly horrifying—and yet this is the narrative technique that allows Halliday as cook (and as daughter) to claim a voice that is her own.

There are two mother figures at the heart of Julie Powell's memoir *Julie & Julia* (2005): the author's own mother, and the towering figure of Julia Child. It is striking that Powell first "conceives" of her project after being told that she has polycystic ovarian syndrome, which may complicate her ability to get pregnant, and is also given a "Pushing Thirty" lecture by her mother (Powell 2005, 12). It is her mother's 1967 edition of Julia Child's *Mastering the Art of French Cooking* that Powell used to peruse often as a child, and it is to Julia Child that Powell turns when she develops the admittedly overambitious project of cooking everything in the volume—and writing about it—back in her tiny kitchen in Queens, where she has a nowhere job as a temp secretary. She brings her mother's copy of Julia Child back to New York with her, and so the project begins.

She remembers finding *The Joy of Sex* in her father's cabinet when she was young, and remarks, "If *The Joy of Sex* was my first taste of sin, *Mastering the Art of French Cooking* was my second" (Powell 2005, 30). As she looked through Julia Child one time and read the sensual, detailed descriptions of such techniques as the creation of pastry dough, she is reminded of that other forbidden book: "Blushing, I shot a glance up at my mom, but she had finished the carrots and was on to the onions" (Powell 2005, 32). Even more, she likes wearing her mother's blue cowl neck sweater while looking at the Julia Child book.

And so it is with this kind of almost overdetermined Freudian set of memories of her parents' sexuality and her own burgeoning sexual awareness that Powell takes the book and begins preparing the French dishes—with her husband Eric, most often, as her spectator and diner. Determined to continue even when the project becomes overwhelming, she has to head off her mother's plea to "*Stop cooking*" (Powell 2005, 43)—as well as what ensues when her mother, whom she describes as a "clean freak" (46), arrives in New York to help her change apartments and shows her "sheer horror" at the state of the place (Powell 2005, 47). At the same time, she realizes that she and her mother share the gift of melodrama, and Powell later recalls the period when her parents were separated because her father was involved with another woman, and Powell would come to school with circles under her eyes as this knowledge weighed upon her. Later, she mentions that the chief tension between her mother and *her* mother—Julie's grandmother—was that the latter was always trying to tell her daughter that she was doing too much: in this sense, Powell remarks, "I figure that Mom, who is terrified above all things of turning into her mother, is reluctant to ride me too hard on this crazy cooking project deal" (Powell 2005, 148). But when Powell goes back to her parents' house in Austin for the holidays, she reports, "My mother did everything short of chaining the kitchen doors shut to keep me from cooking while we were home" (Powell 2005, 153). It takes Powell's childhood friend Isabel to persuade Mrs. Powell that her daughter's project is a worthy one, "And so on the eve of the New Year, I made Veau Prince Orloff for eleven cousins and aunts and uncles, who I'm sure believed their crazy Yankee-fied niece had dropped completely off the deep end" (Powell 2005, 158). Months later, when the project is successfully over, Powell's husband says to her, "If you can do the Project, you can make a kid. No problem" (Powell 2005, 287).

Throughout the memoir, the figure of Julia Child looms large (she was a tall woman), with interspersed fictionalized versions of Child's relationship with her husband and her decision to train as a chef. Strikingly, Child is both a double figure for Powell, and a kind of surrogate mother; after all, she is using her own mother's copy of Child's cookbook, and is attempting to live up to its standards. At the end of the book, it is Powell's mother who calls Powell in tears to tell her that Julia Child has died.

When Powell is finally able to say something about Child's death on her blog, the metaphors of rescue and of the sea show the maternal connection very powerfully: "I have no claim over the woman at all, unless it's the claim one who has nearly drowned has over the person who pulled her out of the ocean" (Powell 2005, 303). And slightly later, she remarks, "Julia taught me what it takes to find your way in the world . . . I thought I was using the Book to learn to cook French food, but really I was learning to sniff out the secret doors of possibility" (Powell 2005, 305–6). Returning to the earlier image of looking secretly at her mother's copy of Julia Child in the same way that she snuck glances at *The Joy of Sex*, these "secret doors" represent the taboo world that the child sees the parents inhabiting; as the child in this case becomes Child (as in Julia Child), Julie/Julia also begins to discover the power of her own subjectivity.

In *Trail of Crumbs: Hunger, Love, and the Search for Home* (2008), memoirist Kim Sunée is largely concerned with loss; in her native country of South Korea, when she was only three years old, her mother abandoned her on a bench in a marketplace, and she was found by the police three days later. The ensuing events are a little hazy in her memory, in part, as she says, because "My adoptive mother keeps changing the story every time I ask her" (Sunée 2008, 2), but she seems to have been taken to an orphanage. She was adopted by an American family and brought to New Orleans, where she was one of only two Asian kids in her school (the other was her sister, who was also adopted), and where she assimilated quickly into Southern American culture. Underlying the memoir, then, is this loss of the mother of whom she has no memory, coupled with the longing to feel a part of her native identity; the end of the chapter about the circumstances of her loss of her mother, for instance, is followed by a kim chi recipe. "My early memories are always related to hunger," she says (Sunée 2008, 7). It is her adoptive grandfather who becomes her closest ally and her cooking mentor (we get his crawfish bisque recipe, for instance); in a sense, he is a mother substitute. Her adoptive mother seems at a loss for how to handle Sunée's approach to womanhood, and Sunée describes the tension between them: "I see her reflection in the mirror—she picks nervously at her worn cuticles, afraid of every day that goes by, watching as my body becomes more like a woman's, my face nowhere near resembling hers. Everything about her is so tightly closed, her life so carefully portioned out" (Sunée 2008, 24). The use of "portion"—a food image—is particularly interesting because throughout the memoir, we get very little association drawn between the adoptive mother and the satisfying of hungers: "I ask my mother what desire means, but she tells me it's like a four-letter word" (Sunée 2008, 25).

At the age of twenty-two, Sunée is swept off her feet by a fabulously wealthy French businessman, who spirits her off to Provence, where she suddenly finds herself in the role of substitute mother to her lover's eight-year-old daughter. During this period of her life, she has very little contact with her family; when she looks at old photos, what she remarks upon is her mother's apparent fear of touching her: "I have the urge to call my family when I look through the photos, but the distance built up over the years is not just geographic" (Sunée 2008, 62). At first, her situation of living a dream existence in Provence is every bit as romantic as it sounds, and Sunée becomes a first-rate French cook as part of her duties in entertaining the many guests who come to their household. The narrative is interspersed with highly seductive-sounding French Provincial recipes, such as "Wild Peaches Poached in Lillet Blanc and Lemon Verbena" (Sunée 2008, xxii). Sunée is resentful when her parents come to visit and her mother asks her with some skepticism if being more or less a kept woman is the way she intends to live her life: "I want her to know that I'm trying as best as I can to invent a life for myself, to discover that there may be a place, no matter how foreign to her, that I can call home" (Sunée 2008, 143). Sunée and her lover travel to Korea and Hong Kong together, though it seems at times as if the trip is almost more for his benefit than for hers, and she becomes very ill by the time that they return to France. Despite his apparent interest in her heritage, however, it soon becomes clear that her lover resents any attempts Sunée makes to discover a creative self by other means such as literature and writing; he expects her to fulfill typically feminine roles of cooking, sex, and nurturing, but not to have further ambitions or to entertain any introspection.

At the end, Sunée has to fight hard to establish an identity of her own as she describes the "fear of waking up with blood in my mouth where someone has cut out my tongue because I have wasted the gift of words. The kitchen is the only place where I am not fearful" (Sunée 2008, 185). She struggles to come to terms with this fear, first by opening her own bookstore, then by seeing an analyst, and eventually by ending the relationship with her lover. When her beloved grandfather dies, she returns to New Orleans and also realizes that even her distance from her mother is something that unites them as they are both reaching for the "intangible parts of the world": she says that "for an instant, I realize how in some ways I do resemble her" (Sunée 2008, 324). It is after further travels, including a trip to French Guiana, that Sunée begins to understand what she wants: "I think about what I've learned in this strange part of the world, about survival and how time has also taught me a lesson—things of the world come when they do, with or without my will" (Sunée 2008, 356). By the end, she even seems to have made peace with the idea of her birth mother as a figure who is both lost and not lost: "I want to one day again brave the South Korean winter in search of a familiar face" (Sunée 2008, 368). Ultimately, she begins to have an understanding of how to merge her multiple cultural identities, which are also her culinary passions—Korean, New Orleansian, French, and now others—into something distinct: "home," she comments, is "in the food that I cook and share with others, in the cities I will come to know . . . " (Sunée 2008, 369).

At the beginning of Laura Schenone's 2008 memoir *The Lost Ravioli Recipes of Hoboken*, she is paying tribute to the memory of her Italian grandparents by making Christmas ravioli; as the author of a previous book about women's historic roles in the kitchen, she is aware of the ironies contained in her behavior as a mother whose children are in the other room: "There was a time when producing great holiday food was an emblem of a mother's skill, her love and generosity . . . But now, there can be little doubt that I am a stubborn and selfish woman for holing up like this on Christmas Day with my back to my family" (Schenone 2008, 8). Throughout the memoir, she confronts these kinds of paradoxes: how can she be a loving mother (and wife and daughter), and yet—a bit like Julie Powell—deal with being overtaken by the need to cook and write obsessively, in the effort to form an identity? She describes her mother as being, a bit like Halliday's mother, "a devoted and eclectic cook who believed in the power of the table, the party, the evening meal. Her repertoire spanned mid- to late-century American—that is to say, heavy on the home economics roasts, iceberg salads, and gelatin molds culled from women's magazines . . . Her cooking was perfectly authentic suburban America, taken up a couple of notches" (Schenone 2008, 14). This is not meant to be an unkind description, and it is certainly one that fits many mothers of Schenone's generation. But the tension comes from Schenone's feeling that she "wanted a deeper food lineage," coming from a family whose varied European ancestors all eventually ended up in Hoboken, of all places. It is by turning to the father—who had always been the more difficult and unreachable family member—and his Italian heritage that Schenone begins to find the focus for her search. She centers this search on tracking down the perfect ravioli recipe, but what she is really doing is finding a way to connect to her elusive father (she calls him a "famously reserved man" [Schenone 2008, 17], and it is his pleasure in some of her pasta-related achievements that seems to give her the most satisfaction.

Her quest is not without its setbacks, including the previously mentioned guilt she feels as a mother over the need to leave her two young sons at various intervals, such as when she makes her first trips to Italy to pursue the recipes and is filled with the pain that she witnesses from them with her departure. She describes the sensation of imagining that a voice is saying to her, "*Get back home to your children*," but couples this with the question of "whether this search for ravioli, this search for the ancient, was really desperation for something beautiful to help me transform the confines of domestic family life?" (Schenone 2008, 61). In the present tense of the story, Schenone's own mother has become very weak from Parkinson's disease, such that she does not even attempt to make the gigantic spread of food that she used to do at Christmas. But one of Schenone's memories is how her formerly very strong mother often had to stand between her children and the father's violent temper: "My mother is the information channel, his publicist and intermediary. When he is quiet, distant, or remiss, she tries to communicate his good intentions. But for decades, my dad is a closed door" (Schenone 2008, 115). She also recognizes her mother's ability to have held her own against her husband's formidable family, citing for example the time that her in-laws thought she was being terribly presumptuous by getting a Bloomingdale's credit card. "It is this faith in family," remarks Schenone, "that gives birth to my mother's elaborate Christmas Eve parties" (Schenone 2008, 163), adding that "She does this for us. She does it for herself. And it nearly kills her each year" (Schenone 2008, 166).

When, at the age of sixteen, Schenone attempted to ask her father about his relationship with her mother and why he felt so entitled to act out his highly patriarchal role, the father is furious and shuts down the conversation completely. Interestingly, though, she also describes this time as a break with her mother: "There always comes a moment when mothers go their own way and daughters walk alone, scattering toward the future in whatever direction they must, like seeds blown off the flowers of a tree" (Schenone 2008, 167). Yet, years later, visiting a family gravesite together brings a hint of Schenone's communion with her mother: "Whenever she is upset or emotional, her Parkinson's flares. We look each other in the eyes, mother and daughter, inextricably linked. When I was a girl, she always told me that I would go to places she never would . . . Whenever this has come true, I have never been able to be purely happy because of my sadness in leaving her behind" (Schenone 2008, 231). At the end of the memoir, Schenone also is able to let go of some of her guilt over abandoning her children at times to work on the project when her oldest son tells her that he, too, wants to learn how to make the ravioli recipes in order to pass them on to his own children some day. As she comments, "Most of us want to pass on something of ourselves" (Schenone 2008, 257)—and in her case, the ravioli seems to contain the secrets of the past and the promise of the future.

Kate Moses' *Cakewalk* (2010) begins in Palo Alto, California, with the image of a mother who resembles Jackie Kennedy and who has three kids under five years old; she had wanted to be an artist, her relentless creativity redirected into "sewing curtains and clothes for our family, gardening, teaching herself to reupholster hand-me-down furniture, concocting elaborate birthday parties and messy art projects for my brothers and me" (Moses 2010, 4). In the opening anecdote, Kate and a neighbor girl get into trouble for eating a cake that the other girl's mother has left out on the counter—and dessert, the longing for sweets, especially cake, becomes the pervading image of the memoir. Her parents stockpile sweet foods and beverages, they eat them at every meal, and she admits that sugar "was the mainstay of my diet as a child" (Moses 2010, 5), but her warring parents never make her feel as if it's okay to take pleasure in it. It's not until she has a son and daughter of her own that she discovers Russell Hoban's Frances books, in which the protagonist is urged to eat and enjoy as much bread and jam (read: cake) as she wants, and Moses realizes how much of her childhood involved a feeling of "furtive criminality" around the idea of sweetness or pleasure (6). The entire memoir, then, becomes about the question of food—particularly cake and other desserts—as connected to needing, wanting, greed, obsession, and withholding.

The mother, who devotes tremendous energy to various scattered creative endeavors, impresses upon her children that they are "heirs to greatness" (Moses 2010, 36), and Moses describes the elaborately detailed birthday cakes that she makes for them. Her childhood is a rollercoaster of maternally generated crests and disappointments, such as when the mother drags her to a department store to try on a Cinderella slipper to win prizes, but makes her so anxious about the ordeal that she throws up and they end up being too late to enter the contest. In first grade, when her family moves to Sonoma, she experiences a crucial moment of independence when the teacher allows her and her classmates to make peanut butter cookies by themselves; for the first time, she realizes that preparing something and having others enjoy eating it can be just as pleasurable as eating it herself. Such moments are rare, though, overwhelmed as she is as a little girl by her mother's volatile and consuming presence.

Moses' father, meanwhile, is distant and preoccupied with his work. He "did not like waste or disorder" (Moses 2010, 40), which of course runs entirely counter to the mother's predilections. She remembers showing up at the dad's law office with her mother holding a picnic basket, but rather than materializing for the picnic (which was meant to celebrate his new job), he sent his secretary out to them with a package of animal cookies, and every time she tried to visit his office from then on—even when he changed law practices—each new secretary would do the same. Her father's unknowability and inaccessibility continues to resonate later in Kate's life.

When the family moves to Pennsylvania—appropriately, to a house on Sugartown Road—one day Kate and her siblings stumble upon an old freezer in the basement that her mother has stocked with a stunning number of snack cakes. Although she says that she later understands her mother's hoarding behavior (which expands as the years go on) as the expression of "unfilled needs" (Moses 2010, 122), at the time, she and her brothers treat the opportunity to sneak an endless number of treats as the fulfillment of long-held cravings: "[f]or once . . . [t]here was plenty of everything for each of us" (Moses 2010, 122). After being bullied at school, Kate becomes convinced that she is fat and hides in the bedroom, eating all of the marshmallows from a box of Lucky Charms. To make matters worse, we learn that the mother is so lonely that she invents excuses to keep Kate home from school, insisting, for example, that she feels a little warm and must have a fever.

While the mother's erratic behavior may have seemed charming when Kate was a child, the older she gets, the more it begins to bother her. When she goes places with them, she so little wants to be associated with being the mother to so many kids that she tells Kate and her siblings to pretend that she is the babysitter: "She only had to tell us once. After the first time, it was a given" (Moses 2010, 157). She has difficulty reconciling the gleeful babysitter role that her mother plays in public with her frequently absent father, compounded by her mother's misguided attempts to take care of her, such as when she has her tonsils out and her mother attempts to administer her penicillin by putting it into the French toast: "I wasn't sure if it was my mom or the babysitter who was taking care of me" (Moses 2010, 160). It's as if she has become accustomed to the idea that her mother plays the roles of two different women, and Kate correspondingly has to know at all times which role she should be playacting. Needless to say, this creates tremendous stress for her, and she suffers from terrible stomach aches as a young adolescent.

The family's subsequent move to Alaska brings out the mother's imbalanced behaviors; she becomes infatuated with the actor McLean Stevenson and tries to get Kate to compose a letter to him pleading that he rescue them from their current "misery and disappointment" (Moses 2010, 176). Even more damaging to Kate is that the mother shows her her secret stash of diet and thyroid pills and Kate, in her desperation to lose weight, begins sneaking pills from her mother's supply whenever she can. In junior high, she realizes that she more or less has the kitchen to herself, as her mother seems at this point to subsist on little else but pills, Tab, and cigarettes, and her brothers fend for themselves. At this point, she finds solace in baking, though she is furious when she makes chocolate chip cookies for a slumber party and her friends, except for Lynn, her closest ally, declare that they have no flavor.

Again and again, the mother tries to transform herself, at one point dragging the fourteen-year-old Kate along with her to a German Club picnic. Kate doesn't want to go—"I didn't want their disgusting sausages. I didn't want the potato salad" (Moses 2010, 195)—but she doesn't really have a choice, and is furious when her mother, who is in a dalliance with the club's president, forces them to spend the night at the picnic ground with the other partiers. She gets a bit of retribution, though, when she fills his beer stein with tadpoles and he unwittingly drinks them. What we see again and again in this narrative is the way that Kate longs for food to be a form of comfort, but in association with her mother, it frequently becomes instead the object of humiliation or anger; at times, she turns this anger inward, and at other times, she enacts revenge through the same medium.

When Kate goes away to college, she eagerly becomes a "sweetheart" of one of the fraternities, but it turns out that this mostly involves doing chores for them—since that includes baking them sugar cookies and other treats, though, she tells herself that she likes it: "I was too busy ministering to the varied appetites and custodial needs of my big brothers to take anything but fleeting notice of how little college resembled what I thought it would be" (Moses 2010, 223). She is also running out of money and spends what little she has on treats like Twinkies, almond candies, and cream pies—in other words, she still uses sugar in an attempt to create some kind of self-nurturing. On a break, she visits her father, who breaks down in tears, saying that he let Kate and her brothers down; this so affects her that when she returns to school, she can't concentrate and ends up in the infirmary with a breakdown, only to hear that her mother thinks she is fabricating her symptoms, and so it is her father who comes to fetch her, with the familiar bag of animal cookies in his hands. The difference, though, is that he is offering them himself rather than putting them into the hands of one of his secretaries. Two of Kate's professors, by encouraging her as a writer, also compensate for the lack of encouragement that she received from her parents. And it's someone else's mother—her boyfriend Peter's mother Nell—who provides a kind of turning point in Kate's relationship with food, as she is a wonderful cook who shares her love of preparing foods from beautiful and fresh ingredients by teaching Kate what she knows. When her mother comes to visit, though, she tries to take credit, saying (upon tasting the eggs that Kate serves her), "I really taught you how to cook, didn't I?" (Moses 2010, 257).

After graduation, when Kate visits her mother in Anchorage, she realizes to her horror that her mother is living like a hoarder, surrounded by bags and piles of stuff in every possible space. When she attempts to cook for her mother and opens the refrigerator, she realizes that even though the fridge is full, everything in it has turned rotten. She tries to help by buying new food, thinking, "[r]egardless of what I might have thought before I arrived—that I no longer needed a mother—my mother still needed me" (Moses 2010, 271). And yet, somewhat predictably, her mother flies into a rage at Kate's efforts to help, screaming at her for throwing out frozen food, which she says *"never* goes bad" (Moses 2010, 272).

Later, when Kate herself becomes a mother, she suffers from postpartum depression—and again, it is surrogate mothering, through a group of other mothers from her aerobics class, that helps her to survive. Her description of her young son's pleasure when he first tastes ice cream allows her to feel a strong connection to him—"Now I know you're mine" (Moses 2010, 321). But being a parent also gives her a different perspective on her own upbringing; she says that motherhood "had taught me that no matter how flawed or inadequate your parents might otherwise be, if they kept you fed and clothed and alive through your first three years, they deserved a lot of credit and no little appreciation" (Moses 2010, 331). Interestingly, though, it's her father, not her mother, to whom she expresses this gratitude in the rest of the paragraph. It is only after her father dies and her mother expresses some remorse about not having been a very good parent that Kate acknowledges the importance of even this small, late level of self-recognition.

In the closing sequence of the memoir, Moses describes the experience, at age forty-five, of impulsively joining a group of grade-schoolers in Golden Gate Park to compete in a cakewalk contest, and to her surprise, they play a song from her childhood—and she is startled to discover that she has won the cake of her choice. She picks the cake that a kindergartener made, flaws and all, covered with sprinkles, "the unmistakable handiwork of someone's cherished child, the proof of love's indulgence" (Moses 2010, 346). It's a beautiful moment as she takes in both the joy of the five-year-old whose cake she has chosen, and her own children congratulating her on having won. The cakewalk of the title, then, is a dance of precariousness, but it is also a tribute to figuring out one's own path to finding sweetness.

One would think from the opening sequences of Gabrielle Hamilton's 2011 memoir *Blood, Bones, and Butter* that her unconventional childhood in a family that threw huge outdoor parties included an ideal, or at least idealized, version of a mother. As a child, Hamilton cherished her mother's French heritage, her past as a ballet dancer, her Hepburn-like eyeliner, and her chic skirts and high heels. More than that, she loved the way her mother had a complete sense of authority in the kitchen and taught them not only to eat exotic cheeses and olives, but even how "to articulate the 's' in salade nicoise and the soup vichysoisse, so that we wouldn't sound like other Americans" (Hamilton 2011, 8). As a young girl, she sits on her mother's lap after dinner every night, goes to the market with her, learns by first grade how to separate chanterelles from poisonous mushrooms.

Her mother's kitchen includes items that other mothers had never even heard of, like a couscoussier, and she "never put a meal together in a careless, eclectic, or incoherent way" (Hamilton 2011, 36). At the time, she didn't fully appreciate her mother's taste in food: for example, "our school lunches were just plain embarrassing: leftover ratatouille, a wedge of Morbier cheese, a bruised pear" (Hamilton 2011, 37). Sometimes, after their baths, she would blindfold Gabrielle and her siblings and spin them around in the fully stocked pantry: "[w]hatever we blinded landed on"— even if it was escargot—"that was our dessert" (Hamilton 2011, 37). From her mother, then, Gabrielle develops a sophisticated palate from a very young age, but her mother's overwhelming personality dominates the kitchen.

It is not until her parents' marriage begins to fall apart that she begins to have a sense of her mother's unhappiness and anger: she sees her mother's eyes after a blowout fight, and thinks, "*What a fucking bitch*" (Hamilton 2011, 26), yet is thrown for a loop when her mother announces casually at a family meeting that she and the five kids (though the kids were never actually consulted on this) have decided that the father needs to leave. And the following summer, her mother moves to a remote part of Vermont—and since the father is preoccupied with financial issues, Gabrielle (at the age of thirteen) and her siblings are more or less left to fend for themselves, a situation that today, she remarks, would have ended in someone calling Child Services. At that age, her opportunities for work are limited, but she gets a job washing dishes at a local restaurant, and "that, just like that, is how a whole life can start" (Hamilton 2011, 34). In retrospect, she says, there probably would have been some adults who would have given her more "purpose and direction" (Hamilton 2011, 35), but she spends her time around ones who are fascinated by the way, with her swearing and her "red tube top" (Hamilton 2011, 36), she's acting more mature than she really is. But as the result of these jobs—and more than that, being left alone to forage in her mother's once-ample pantry, she remarks, "During this summer, I learned to cook. I spent most of my time in our home in the kitchen, opening old jars of stuff my mother had left behind" (Hamilton 2011, 36).

Hamilton eventually makes her way through college (on the third try) and attends graduate school in writing at the University of Michigan, all while working in many different restaurant kitchens and ultimately becoming the celebrated chef-owner of Prune in New York City. What is somewhat shocking, though, is that her mother drops out of the memoir entirely for many pages—during which Hamilton herself becomes a mother—and when she reappears in chapter 14, we get an almost-casual mention that they have not seen one another in twenty years. Her explanation of this, or lack of explanation, is poignant: "She was, wasn't she, the very heartbeat of the most cherished period of my life? So what is there to make of the simplistic thing I've come to utter in explanation . . . I feel better without her" (Hamilton 2011, 174–75).

After her brother Todd dies suddenly of a stroke, though, Hamilton decides to bring her husband and baby with her to visit her mother, but the anticipation of the visit is almost worse than the visit itself. She coaches her Italian husband that he will only be able to take five-minute showers and so forth: "My mother's frugality can be so acute that it takes on an actual hostility" (Hamilton 2011, 178). In her dread of the visit, she even compares her mother to a black widow spider, saying that with her "certain poisoning, I am thirteen all over again" (Hamilton 2011, 180).

And yet, when they arrive, Gabrielle is stunned that her mother has made an elegant dinner and has even made two roast chickens when one would have sufficed. Touchingly, her mother is modest about the food: "She makes apologies to me, her chef daughter, in advance of the meal even though I am certain we both know that I learned to cook, exclusively, from her" (Hamilton 2011, 182). But when she awakens the next morning and realizes that her mother is spying on her and her husband through the window curtains, the black widow spider imagery returns as she depicts her mother "rubbing her six hairy legs together with hungry impatience, for hours" (Hamilton 2011, 184).

A turning point comes, though, when she sees how age and time have ravaged her mother, as she views this woman who once wore eyeliner every morning peering at them through the window with two pairs of glasses on. She longs, in effect, for her mother to really see her—to "observe that I had become something of a full-fledged, self-possessed adult with rights and wishes regarding her affections" (Hamilton 2011, 187). Instead, though, she notices that her always impossibly chic French mother is wearing Payless shoes with rubber bands holding up her socks—and more than that, she's kind of proud to be doing so, since the sensible shoes were such a bargain. The sight of this fills Gabrielle with fear that she will turn out the same way in her old age, and she tries to recover the moment by turning their conversation to talk about food and wine. Even then, the conversation is freighted by the discovery that her mother, who had always seemed such a worldly cook, wants to know how the *tom yum* soup paste that Gabrielle brought is used: "Is it possible that I now know more than she does about food and cooking? Have I surpassed her?" (Hamilton 2011, 190). This leads her to wonder exactly what it was that happened that made her distance herself from her mother for twenty years. On some level, she understands that when she was a child, her family's difference from other families was something that was "arduously protected . . . Most people ate Mrs. Paul's frozen fish sticks and Kraft macaroni and cheese and Oscar Mayer bologna, but we ate coq au vin, sesame bread sticks, and le puy lentils for less money than the store-bought stuff" (Hamilton 2011, 191–92). While these may sound like memories to cherish, Gabrielle also feels that she was forced to internalize the message that her family was somehow better, and has spent twenty years resenting what she calls "Gallic snobbery" (Hamilton 2011, 192).

When, in the present, though, she sees her mother mixing jug wine and blackberry schnapps—effectively, a cheap wine cooler—as her preferred beverage, something in her gives way and "the oppressive heavy wet burden of snow slides off the roof of my soul in one giant thawing chunk and suddenly I feel clear, light, and permissive" (Hamilton 2011, 192). Even though, as Gabrielle and her husband and child prepare to leave, she says that she still feels uncomfortable when her mother touches her, something essential has changed: as she sees that her mother's impossible standards have relaxed, it feels like a breakthrough for her to realize that she herself can let go of the tension she has created—"these perfectionisms, elitisms, excellences" (Hamilton 2011, 192)—over the years.

Diana Abu-Jaber's 2005 memoir *The Language of Baklava* and its sequel, *Life without a Recipe* (2016), differ from these other "angry daughter" memoirs because most of the attention is directed toward the father rather than the mother. Abu-Jaber was raised by her Jordanian father, Bud, an extremely volatile, passionate, and funny character who was also the primary cook in her family, and by her American mother; various aunts, uncles, and other relatives on both sides of the family—especially Grace, her mother's mother—play strong roles as well. As a child, Abu-Jaber lived alternately in the United States and in Jordan, and as a result, she both fits and does not fit into the two cultures. Her father, who "learns English not from books but from soaking in the language of work, of the shops and restaurants" (Abu-Jaber 2005, 2), loves cooking, dreams of one day owning his own restaurant, and tests guests and suitors by offering them food.

Strikingly, Abu-Jaber's American mother is a harder figure to get to know in the two memoirs, in part at least because her presence is overwhelmed by Bud's larger-than-life one, and in part because her method of dealing with her husband's impulsive (and sometimes irrational) plans is to go along with (or sometimes act as if she is going along with) them. His older sister, Abu-Jaber's Auntie Aya, is the only one who seems to exert some sort of authority over Bud. And when Diana, as a teenager, confesses her anger and confusion about her Jordanian-American identity, it is Auntie Aya who—through the act of making baklava—teaches her that food is intimately connected to one's gender and culture, but perhaps not in the ways one expects. The revelatory moments begin when Auntie Aya says that given the choice of a baby or cake, she always chose cake: "this is the first intimation I've heard of another way through life" (Abu-Jaber 2005, 186). Auntie Aya tells Diana that the complex emotions that food generates are not all about simple pleasure, especially considering the gendered history of its preparation; she says, "Food is aggravation and too much work and hurting your back and trapping the women inside like slaves" (Abu-Jaber 2005, 189). The critical moment comes when Auntie Aya invites Diana to taste the baklava and to consider how doing so constitutes an acknowledgment of multiple cultures (since it is Arabic, Turkish, Greek, etc.) and is therefore an act of *listening*. Auntie Aya says, "I looked, I tasted, I spoke kindly and truthfully, I invited. You know what else? I keep doing it" (Abu-Jaber 2005, 190). And when Diana tries the baklava herself and realizes that it is "like a poem" (Abu-Jaber 2005, 191), she also experiences a moment later that evening, when her father joins them in eating it, of "recognition" about the idea of "home" (Abu-Jaber 2005, 192).

The other powerful female figure in Abu-Jaber's life is Grace, or Gram, her mother's mother, who is at least as strong-willed as Bud, though in very different ways. Her cooking style is traditional older-generation American—when she first meets her daughter's future husband, she can't understand why his dietary laws forbid him from eating ham, and Abu-Jaber includes her Sunday roast beef recipe that is basically meat with salt and pepper put in the oven to roast. She thrives on buying candy for her grandchildren, giving them shot glasses full of M&Ms and allowing them to load the grocery cart with any kind of candy they desire. The funniest chapter in *The Language of Baklava* is about when Gram brings a young Diana to an Asian ("Oriental") restaurant in New York City and proceeds to embarrass Diana greatly when she engages in conversation with their elderly Chinese waiter. Having been betrayed by her late husband, Gram harbors an insatiable hatred of men. As we see in *Life without a Recipe*, wherein memories of Gram return frequently, her advice to Diana is: "Never learn how to sew, cook, type, or iron . . . That's how they get you" (Abu-Jaber 2016, 18). Like Auntie Aya (with whom Gram eventually has a long-distance friendship), Gram represents a powerful force for Diana. Again, her influence is not a maternal one, but rather, it gives her an alternate source of strength and equips her for making decisions that are independent of the ones that her father wants her to make.

When Diana goes away to college, she goes through a period where she subsists on candy and becomes physically ill every time that she returns home and tries to eat the traditional Jordanian dishes that her father has prepared; she acknowledges it as a "rejection of something more powerful than food" (Abu-Jaber 2005, 227). Then, one night, she awakes to an image of a purple light "like a benediction" (Abu-Jaber 2005, 229) that allows her to feel the connections between people, between America and Jordan, and her hunger for the food of her heritage finally returns, though it is fascinating that in describing the redemption of the moment, she goes to the fridge and eats *lebeneh* (yogurt) with pita bread, saying, "Tonight, this is the purest food in the world. Mother's milk" (Abu-Jaber 2005, 229). In a sense, she has allowed herself to be remothered by her father, but to do so on her own terms. And again, her mother is more or less absent from this scene.

The Language of Baklava ends with Abu-Jaber's declaration that she is a "Bedouin" (Abu-Jaber 2005, 327) who must make her way out into the world. In *Life without a Recipe*, the theme of parenthood becomes even more complicated as she not only faces her father's old age and declining heath, but she herself becomes a mother. In her narrative of adopting Grace, her baby daughter (named for her grandmother), she learns that mothering is largely an act of improvisation. She says that if she could, she would have asked Auntie Aya for a description of the steps toward gaining courage, but then realizes that such steps couldn't be written down: "You had to do it by feel" (Abu-Jaber 2016, 263).

A discussion of mothers in recent food memoirs would not be complete without including a consideration of the work of Ruth Reichl. In *Tender at the Bone* and *Comfort Me with Apples,* the first two volumes of her wonderful three-part memoir (the third, *Garlic and Sapphires,* is mostly about Reichl's adventures as a *New York Times* restaurant critic), the mother is a prominent character who shaped Reichl's relationship with food, and in her short later book *For You Mom, Finally* (which is not really a food memoir, though food is always present), she attempts to come to terms with her mother's deeply held frustrations. Reichl explains in this later volume that she is grateful not to have been born in her mother's generation, in what she calls "the worst possible time to have been a middle-class American woman" (Reichl 2010, 7). Her mother was a brilliant woman whose desire to become a doctor was thwarted by her parents, who forced her to study music instead, and she was part of the generation of women who were expected to marry and have kids rather than pursuing their own careers. As she was growing up, Reichl could see her mother's incredible unhappiness and her lack of outlets for her creative energy:

> [B]y the time Mom married so many labor-saving devices had been introduced that cooking and cleaning just didn't take that long. My mother, like most of her friends, literally had nothing to do . . . It was a terrible waste of talent and energy, and watching them I knew that I was never going to be like them . . . I realized that [my father's] secret life, the one he had away from us, nurtured him, fed his soul. I watched him leaving in the morning, wishing that my mother could go to work too. I thought if she had her own secret life she would be a happier person. And I determined, when I was very small, that no matter what, nobody was going to keep me from having a work life. I thought then—and I still think now—that it is the key to happiness. (Reichl 2010, 9–10)

We learn early on in *Tender at the Bone* that the mother's experiments with leftovers and bargain food sometimes have results perilous to guests' health, and that Reichl as a child frequently had to warn guests and relatives (behind her mother's back, of course) not to eat the things they were served: that the sour cream on St. Patrick's Day, for example, was green not because of food coloring but because it had been in the fridge for too long. She says that these experiences taught her "that food could be dangerous, especially to those who loved it. I took this very seriously. My parents entertained a great deal, and before I was ten I had appointed myself guardian of the guests" (Reichl 1998, 5). The many passages in which Reichl describes her mother's peculiar relationship with food are both amusing to the reader, and heartbreaking when we consider how much Reichl as a child had to take on as a result. Interestingly, in her later book *For You Mom, Finally*, Reichl expresses some chagrin about the way that after her first two memoirs were published, people often asked her with some incredulity whether her mother really did the outlandish things she describes; she says that while everything is true, she never would have told these stories while her mother was still alive, and even so, "[a]lthough I omitted the most embarrassing tales, the first time I held the printed book in my hands I winced" because she felt that she had betrayed her mother and wanted (by means of this later book) to "make it right" (Reich 2010, 5).

What we come to realize in the first memoir is that the mother is clinically manic-depressive, and Reichl includes many descriptions of the parties where the mother's half-abandoned ideas go out of control—including an engagement party at which most of the guests end up with food poisoning. According to Reichl, "Most mornings I got out of bed and went to the refrigerator to see how my mother was feeling. You could tell instantly just by opening the door. One day in 1960 I found a whole suckling pig staring at me . . . This was not a bad sign: the more odd and interesting things there were in the refrigerator, the happier my mother was likely to be" (Reichl 1998, 8). As a child, she longs for the normalcy of her friends' mothers, a theme that we see in so many of these memoirs. Her friend Jeanie's mother "served the sort of perfect lunches that I longed for: neat squares of cream cheese and jelly on white bread, bologna sandwiches, Chef Boyardee straight from the can" (Reichl 1998, 9).

Reichl attributes her own passion for cooking to the lessons she received from relatives and housekeepers who nurtured her in the absence of her mother's ability to do so, as well as to her need to claim a sense of reliability and independent accomplishment. She says, "Unknowingly I had started sorting people by their tastes. Like a hearing child born to deaf parents, I was shaped by my mother's handicap, discovering that food could be a way of making sense of the world" (Reichl 1998, 6). These other women, early on, become surrogate mothers to the largely unmothered Ruth, and impart to her their love for food. Her Aunt Birdie's housekeeper, Alice, for example, is a key influence. Reichl calls her "the first person I ever met who understood the power of cooking. She was a great cook, but she cooked more for herself than for other people, not because she was hungry but because she was comforted by the rituals of the kitchen" (Reichl 1998, 26). This emphasis on "rituals" and on "comfort" plays precisely to the two things that Ruth doesn't receive from her own mother. As she follows Alice to the markets and watches her conversing with the merchants, asking them questions, Ruth says that she "began to see the status conferred by caring about food" (Reichl 1998, 27).

Another substitute mother figure in Ruth's childhood is the house-keeper Mrs. Peavey, who had a "patrician manner" and "spoke three languages fluently" (Reichl 1998, 36); she refuses Mrs. Reichl's request for a sweet potato marshmallow casserole at Thanksgiving, calling it a "horrid middle-class concoction" (Reichl 1998, 38). We find out that Mrs. Peavey seems to have a drinking problem, and after she doesn't show up for a few days, Ruth volunteers to her mother (who won't get out of bed) to make wiener schnitzel; with a sense of accomplishment, she buys the ingredients by herself, and then Mrs. Peavey shows up to help her, announcing at the end of this interaction that she is leaving the Reichl household to become a cook. Mrs. Peavey's parting advice to Ruth, which she takes to heart, is to look out for herself rather than letting others tell her how to live her life—and always (in a reference to an earlier household incident) to make extra pastry for the Beef Wellington.

Throughout *Tender at the Bone* and *Comfort Me with Apples*, Reichl is torn between a sense of wanting to be stable like her father (her first husband eerily resembles her father, as she soon realizes), and echoing her mother's wild creativity. Ultimately, the mother is both a figure from whom Reichl needs to get away (thus her move to California), and one whose illness and eccentricity she attempts to embrace: "Being a family meant dealing with Mom" (Reichl 1998, 248). Even as she begins to become successful in her career, her mother's real or imagined voice haunts her, leading her to have panic attacks. Her success as a food writer somehow does not win her the approval from her mother that she so longs for: "'Food!' said my mother disdainfully. 'All you do is write about food.' I tried to get my mother's voice out of my head, but it was always there" (Reichl 1998, 269). Sometimes she imagines that a "phantom" version of her mother is before her eyes, scolding her, for example, for an expensive meal at Guy Savoy in Paris. Her mother's presence still haunts her at every turn, yet the key change is that she is also learning to silence that imaginary voice:

> Though uninvited, my mother appeared with the first course. "Is this how you will spend the next ten days?" she inquired. "Eating absurdly expensive food all by yourself? Trying to impress waiters? Where will the money come from?"
>
> "Be quiet, please," I said. "I'm busy. I want to remember every detail of this soup." (Reichl 2001, 37)

This moment, the argument with the phantom mother, makes an apt image for all of the writers I've talked about here. Anger at the mother, in a certain way, drives the daughter and urges her on in her pursuit of exquisite cuisine, of finding a different palate, or of finding a different culinary world to inhabit. And yet she is always also in some kind of a dialogue with the mother, even when the latter is absent. The mother is both muse and nemesis, the first provider of food for the daughter, but also the direct cause of the daughter's later need to rebel, to find her own voice and her own palate. When the daughter eats, the mother—sometimes chiding, and sometimes nurturing—is never sitting very far away.

SEVEN

Eat and Run

Food Writing, Masculinity, and the "Male Midlife Crisis"

In the previous chapter, I discussed the topic of "angry daughters" in several recent food memoirs written by women. Later, though, I began thinking about the question of whether the food memoir in its contemporary form deserves to be considered, again through the lens of gender studies, as a genre that takes on issues of being a son rather than a daughter, a man in the wake of a crisis like a divorce, a man preoccupied with questions of sexuality, body image, or just plain hunger. My intention here is to examine these issues through a range of men's food memoirs by professional chefs, food critics, dramatists, and journalists (Anthony Bourdain, Jonathan Reynolds, Bob Spitz, Frank Bruni, and Marcus Samuelsson). In one of the many commercials for erectile dysfunction drugs that ran on television not too long ago, a chic-looking African-American woman gives her man a meaningful look as they sit at the table together, and they go upstairs. But just when you think the obvious is about to happen, we see them on their way back downstairs, now all dressed up and on their way out to dinner. The promise of this particular drug is that the man will be ready any time—but the suggestion of the commercial is that the fancy restaurant meal has to happen first. Eating is foreplay, but it is also a transaction, a contract, and a potential source of anxiety, sexual and otherwise.

In her history of cookbooks in American culture, Megan J. Elias talks about the "gendering" of the male gourmet, pointing out that when *Gourmet* magazine was first created in 1941, the target audience was men, not women, and its rhetoric attempted to distance the publication from others that focused on women as the primary cooks, or as Elias puts it, "[i]n order to get men into the kitchen . . . women's longstanding dominance had to be overturned" (Elias 2017, 97). One writer, Walter Buehr, conveyed his disdain for feminine tearoom-like establishments and celebrated the "red-blooded extravert [*sic*]" who enjoyed watching meat cook; both the editorial content and the ads were aimed at middle-class men. Another *Gourmet* writer, Eric Howard, insisted, "Women are good cooks, but it is axiomatic that men are better. Women are inclined to follow recipes too closely. They may be adept at complicated desserts, tricky salads . . . but much of their cooking is fussy and finicky . . . women do not cook, generally, with the fine careless rapture of the male" (Elias 2017, 97). The attempt to create a masculinized version of the gourmet cook marks a fascinating moment in American culture, particularly as it reveals the gap between stereotypes of the home cook (principally female) and the restaurant chef (principally male).

Although the food memoir has recently been stereotyped as a women's genre (with works like *Julie and Julia* and *Eat, Pray, Love* becoming best sellers and feature films), literary/cultural scholars pursuing issues of masculinity (anxiety, aging, competition, homosociality, etc.) would be fascinated to discover that there is indeed a substantive number of recent creative nonfiction books on food by male authors. The confessional approach—one that uses food to explore the undercurrents of the writer's emotional life—becomes the focus of a surprising number of these texts. I would like to discuss what I will call the "male mid-life crisis food memoir," in which—for all of these works—the creation and the resolution of a challenge to the middle-aged author's masculinity comes about through cooking and eating.

When Anthony Bourdain took his own life in June 2018, it sent powerful reverberations of shock and sorrow throughout not only the world of his fellow chefs, but also through the huge audience who knew him for his irreverent food books, his appearances as a judge on cooking competition shows like *Top Chef* and *The Taste*, and for the various travel/food series (*No Reservations, Parts Unknown*) which he hosted on The Travel Channel and more recently on CNN. Tributes from fans and longtime friends from the culinary world poured in. Eric Ripert wrote, "Anthony was my best friend. An exceptional human being, so inspiring and generous. One of the great storytellers who connected with so many" (Campbell-Schmitt 2018). Andrew Zimmern commented, "Tony was a symphony. I wish everyone could have seen all of him" (Campbell-Schmitt 2018). Jose Andrés said, addressing him posthumously, "[Y]ou only saw beauty in all people[;] you will always travel with me" (Campbell-Schmitt). And Ruth Reichl lamented, "Oh Tony. Oh no. Sitting here weeping. There will never be another like you. Really tragic loss" (Campbell-Schmitt 2018). This is just a small sampling of the vast number of heartfelt responses to

Bourdain's unexpected death at the age of sixty-one, but these words don't tell the full story of Bourdain's unexpected journey from a celebrator of all things macho about the world of cuisine to an eloquent defender of women's rights not to be sexually harassed in the kitchen or elsewhere.

Bourdain first generated mass public attention in 2000 while he was the executive chef at Les Halles in New York City and published the influential book *Kitchen Confidential*, which exposes many of the secrets of the restaurant industry: don't order the fish special on a Monday because it is probably made from unsold goods about to go bad and disguised by a sauce; the rolls in your breadbasket have probably been taken out of a previous diner's breadbasket; avoid the Hollandaise sauce at brunch because it has been sitting out and is probably full of bacteria—and so forth. More than that, though, *Kitchen Confidential* offers an inside look at the machismo of the restaurant kitchen and a startlingly frank vision of the physical toll that the supposedly glamorous life of a chef actually exacts upon someone who aspires to this career. On the one hand, I wouldn't strictly call this a "male midlife crisis" memoir, since it in some ways prefaces and creates the further acting-out of that crisis in Bourdain's later books like *A Cook's Tour* and *The Nasty Bits*. But this famously testosterone-laden account of a life spent in restaurant kitchens where there is an entire set of codes for masculine behavior has a huge influence on the other authors' books that followed.

The first section of the book is the most memoirlike, containing an account of how Bourdain, as a child forced to summer with his parents in the French countryside, was initially a fussy eater—but his first taste of vichysoisse taught him that food "could be *important*. It could be an event. It had secrets" (Bourdain 2000, 13). Furious after his parents leave him and his brother in the car while they go to a three-hour French meal, Bourdain seeks his revenge by outdoing the rest of his family in his willingness to try new foods: "Stinky, runny cheeses that smelled like dead men's feet? Horsemeat? Sweetbreads? Bring it on!! Whatever had the most shock value became my meal of choice" (Bourdain 2000, 13). This culminates in his tasting his first oyster, which he characterizes as having the significance of a sexual initiation: "I remember it like I remember losing my virginity—and in many ways, more fondly" (Bourdain 2000, 14). A later piece about his childhood in *Medium Raw* also characterizes childhood anger—in this case, at having a relatively "normal" family when he envied the kids whose parents let them roam wildly: "I envied them their dysfunctional and usually empty houses, their near-total lack of supervision" (Bourdain 2010, 20).

Even his introduction to cooking, which occurs in a series of summer jobs in Provincetown, is all about the feeling of male power that he derives from the experience. Not only does he say he first realized he wanted to be a chef when he sees the bride from a wedding at the restaurant sneak out of the reception to have sex with one of the cooks, but he sees a direct connection between doing such jobs as manning the broiler and exercising masculine prowess:

> I cannot describe to you the sheer pleasure, the *power* of commanding that monstrous, fire-breathing iron and steel furnace, bumping the grill under the flames with my hip the way I'd seen Bobby and Jimmy do it. It was tremendous. I couldn't have felt happier—or more powerful—in the cockpit of an F-16. (Bourdain 2000, 30)

His pleasure in becoming a line cook gets depicted as a form of male sexual conquest: "I was a line stud, an all-around guy, a man's man" (Bourdain 2000, 117). Throughout the book, Bourdain unabashedly uses masculine metaphors—boxing, having a boner, etc.—to characterize the scuffles and excitement of working in a restaurant kitchen. He argues that cooks who consider themselves "artists" are "geared more to giving themselves a hard-on" than to making customers happy (Bourdain 2000, 63). A successful tower of chicken breast and mashed potatoes looms "like a fully engorged Priapus over my awed and cowering guests"; the hyperbole is of course deliberately and amusingly provocative, but he's also showing us the absolute phallocentrism of the restaurant kitchen (Bourdain 2000, 78).

When he's interviewing for a new job and tells the owners that he does food that is simply prepared from the best ingredients, he offers the aside that what he is communicating is that "there was something less than masculine—even gay—about dressing a hunk of meat up like a goddamn birthday cake" (Bourdain 2000, 159). When he and his sous-chef Steven (a pseudonym) are looking for personnel to add to their lineup at a new restaurant, he says that they "*raped* every kitchen we could think of" (Bourdain 2000, 170; Bourdain's italics). Sports and military imagery prevail. He characterizes the discussion of an evening's dinner service at the end of the night as "postgame analysis" but he also conflates this with a Vietnam image: "We're gonna fight Dien Bien Phu over and over again every night. I don't care if we lose the war—we're *professionals*, man. We're the motherfuckin' *A-Team*, the pros from Dover, cool breeze . . . " (Bourdain 2000, 215). When he describes what he wants his runners to be like, he mentions both "that rabid, pregame, caged-animal mentality one looks for in a professional fullback" and that he wants his "runners hyperventilating like Marines about to take a hill before the rush comes" (Bourdain 2000, 228). There is an entire chapter in *Kitchen Confidential*—a fascinating one—on the masculinist language used by chefs. "It's all about dick, you see," he says, and goes on to describe how what he calls the "real international language of cuisine" involves playing the dozens (an old game of trading insults) in the most phallocentric and homosocial way possible; he notes, "All comments must, out of historical necessity, concern involuntary rectal penetration, penis size, physical flaws or annoying mannerisms or defects" (Bourdain

2000, 220). He professes admiration for female line cooks when they are tough enough to play with the big boys: "To have a tough-as-nails, foul-mouthed, trash-talking female line cook on your team can be a true joy—and a civilizing factor in a unit where conversation tends to center around [*sic*] who's got the bigger balls and who takes it in the ass" (Bourdain 2000, 58).

To a certain degree, what we can see in *Kitchen Confidential* is the male midlife crisis in preparation as it is about to cook up. Such chapters as "A Day in the Life" describe what Bourdain puts himself through, at the peak of his success as executive chef of New York City's Les Halles and its sister restaurants, in a typical day. At this point he has kicked some more serious drug problems (frankly admitting to having had a heroin addiction), but has to function with a maniacal amount of energy to get through the multitasking necessary to run a high-end dining establishment. He describes having the bartender make him a beer stein-sized margarita partway through dinner service and says, "The drink manages to take the edge off my raging adrenaline buzz and goes down nicely after the three double espressos, two beers, three cranberry juices, eight aspirins, two ephedrine drinks and a hastily gobbled hunk of merguez, which I managed to squeeze into a heel of bread before swallowing in two bites" (Bourdain 2000, 198).

This kind of life proved not to be sustainable, but what Bourdain did was to parlay his experience with food, combined with his pleasure at part-time writing (he published *Bone in the Throat*, a cooking-based murder mystery), into an enviable gig as a travel writer and TV food journalist—a step we see him taking near the end of *Kitchen Confidential*. Near the beginning of *A Cook's Tour*, he even makes fun of the success of that book, saying, "I'd just put down a very nice score with an obnoxious and overtestosteroned account of my life in the restaurant business. Inexplicably, it had flown off the shelves" (Bourdain 2001, 5). And he explains that he uses the leverage of the book's success to explain to his editor that he wants something more: adventure, travel, magic. On the one hand, this shift marked a typical midlife crisis as he threw aside everything (including, eventually, his first and second marriages) to travel the world tasting various exotic cuisines and writing about them (in books such as *A Cook's Tour*) as well as establishing a wider reputation as an adventurer on his TV shows such as *No Reservations*. "Survival has its costs," he says, in reference to a chef friend, but he could just as easily have been talking about himself (Bourdain 2000, 246). "We are all the stars of our own private movie," he remarks in the book that was designed to accompany his *No Reservations* show: "heroic, tragically misunderstood, and of course, much more sympathetic than we are in real life" (Bourdain 2007, 282).

We even see him, in *The Nasty Bits*, trying to convince Gabrielle Hamilton to write her own book (which is probably what turned into *Blood,*

Bones, & Butter, discussed in the previous chapter) "I attempt to convince her to write the women's version of *Kitchen Confidential*. 'You'd make me look like a freakin' manicurist!' I insist. 'This is a book that *needs to be written*. Isn't there *enough* testosterone in this genre?'" (Bourdain 2006, 84–85). In many moments of the pieces in his 2010 *Medium Raw*, we see him express self-doubt and second thoughts (though, paradoxically, still presented with a certain swagger) about the success and some of the content of *Kitchen Confidential*. In his preface, he describes sitting at a tableful of renowned fellow chefs and asks, "What could my memoir of an undistinguished—even disgraceful—career have said to people of such achievements?" (Bourdain 2010, xviii). He has an entire essay in *Medium Raw* called "The Fish-on-Monday Thing" which he begins by saying, "I was genuinely angry most mornings, writing *Kitchen Confidential*" (Bourdain 2010, 254), explaining that his anger was fueled by overwork and financial anxiety, as well as a failing marriage and a recent attempt to kick his drug addiction. He adds that the real anger he was experiencing while composing the memoir turned out to be the attitude, once the book was published, that most people expected from him. Though he claims still to feel an antipathy towards vegetarians, he backpedals a bit on some of his denunciations of TV chefs. At the end of the piece, he calls himself a "cranky old fuck" and says that he's still angry, but that we should go ahead and "*eat* the fucking fish on Monday already" and that his customers, who at the time he wrote the first memoir, were the biggest subjects of his anger, are no longer a target (Bourdain 2010, 268). In an interview with Elvis Mitchell published as an afterword to the book, he tells Mitchell that he saw *Medium Raw* as largely being about "the disconnect between what my life was like when I wrote *Kitchen Confidential* and what my life is like now" (Mitchell 2010, 4).

To some degree, part of Bourdain's appeal was this ability to mock himself for becoming the kind of celebrity food professional upon whom he previously heaped abuse; he says, "My hands, which I'm so proud of in the final pages [of *Kitchen Confidential*], are soft and lovely now—like a little baby girl's. I suck. I comfort myself that I was reaching the end of my usefulness as a line cook anyway" (Bourdain 2000, xv). But there was clearly also a kind of disingenuousness at work at this point, since the next phase of Bourdain's career also caused him to serve as a kind of fantasy figure or bad-boy role model for those who would envision a life that contains such moments as eating snakes for a TV audience. Another side of him, a more unabashedly sentimental and introspective one, emerges at moments like the closing paragraphs of the *No Reservations* book, when he reflects on the return home after each exotic journey and describes watching his baby daughter sleep—an especially evocative choice since (a) he is talking about a daughter rather than a son, and (b) in the line cited above, he had self-deprecatingly described his own hands as being like a baby girl's. Here, though, he says that as he sees "her expression changing second by second as pleasure, fear, concern, and wonder flash across her brain, I find . . . something." He explains that he has "seen those expressions elsewhere and everywhere. Maybe the differences between places are no less—and no more—pronounced than the distance between human hearts" (Bourdain 2007, 285).

Bourdain's girlfriend, actress Asia Argento, was one of many women who accused movie mogul Harvey Weinstein of sexual assault—leading to what become known as the #MeToo movement in which many men, including quite a few in positions of public prominence, were outed for sexual misconduct. This put Bourdain, with all of the macho rhetoric of works like *Kitchen Confidential*, in a tricky position. To his credit, though, it marked what might be called the second midlife crisis point for him, as he began to take a fierce and self-implicating look at his own persona. As Adam Campbell-Schmitt writes in his summary of the responses to Bourdain's suicide, "In his later years, he would become outspoken on many issues, both political and professional, including the toxic workplace he wrote about and how that environment fosters the sexual harassment and assault most recently brought to light by the #MeToo movement" (Campbell-Schmitt 2018). Kat Kinsman, who eventually became friends with Bourdain after years of verbal warfare, eloquently characterizes Bourdain's late change of heart:

> For a while, he cared about heroin and other excesses, but then he didn't seem to anymore in recent years. Still, that fixed him in the heads of many people—especially those drawn to kitchens—as a nihilistic rock star, bad boy, hard-driving pirate captain who saw self-abuse and workaholism as a badge of honor, and they did their damnedest to emulate him. But even Bourdain was past that these days and expressed tremendous regret at the "meathead" culture that had metastasized out of his chronicle of kitchen life, *Kitchen Confidential*. He spoke precisely and passionately about the failings of the industry—his own included—and the culture at large. He named names, he poked hives, he charged at mountains. (Kinsman 2018)

And most tellingly, in his self-confrontation, Bourdain had to admit that due to his past posturing, there were reasons that women "did not come to him to talk about such things" (Gajanan 2018). In a number of interviews, he talked about his own past complicity, saying on *The Daily Show* in January 2018, for instance, "I came out of a brutal, oppressive business that was historically unfriendly to women . . . I knew a lot of women, it turned out, who had stories about their experiences—about people I know—who did not feel I was the sort of person they could confide in" (Gajanan 2018). And in an interview with *Slate* in October 2017, he was even more direct:

> I am a guy on TV who sexualizes food. Who uses bad language. Who thinks our discomfort, our squeamishness, fear and discomfort around

matters sexual is funny. I have done stupid offensive shit . . . And because I was a guy in a guy's world who had celebrated a system—I was very proud of the fact that I had endured that. (Gajanan 2018)

The later parts of Bourdain's story, then, mark an attempt to come to terms with his past with the same refreshing honesty and bluntness evident in his writing (and in his TV persona) all through his career. While he seemed to have had everything, it's well-known by now that no one, no matter how famous or successful, is exempt from a mental health crisis. We'll never know exactly what the circumstances were that led Bourdain to take his own life, or even whether it was fully a deliberate act. It's a true tragedy that eventually, his intertwined biological and psychological demons were too much for him.

Wrestling with Gravy (2006) is critic and dramatist Jonathan Reynolds's account of how his upper-crust childhood and later troubled relationships were always intermingled with food. Reynolds has been a moderately successful screenwriter (*Micki and Maude* and other films in the 1980s) and playwright (*Stonewall Jackson's House*—a Pulitzer nominee—and *Geniuses*), and for five years wrote a food column for the *New York Times Magazine*. The early parts of his memoir emphasize how both traumas and celebrations in his life were always connected with food; just as Bourdain's earliest memory that food was "important" came when he tasted vichyssoise on the boat to France, Reynolds's transatlantic crossing on the France as a youth was transformative: "What happened next redirected my life. I sat down to eat" (Reynolds 2006, 75). Yet food memories for him, far more than for Bourdain, are also sometimes connected with grief; for example, he says that to this day, he can't have a meal in Paris without remembering the time he was there with his girlfriend and his distant, wealthy father—and his father ended up propositioning his girlfriend.

Perhaps not surprisingly, Reynolds begins to see the cultivation of skills as a cook as a means, sometimes a misleading one, of attaining the feeling that it is something he can oversee even when the rest of his life is falling apart. He insists, "Food is controllable, while most of life isn't. And cooking is power. If you're the chef, you're determining what people eat" (Reynolds 2006, x). He adds, "I cook most when feeling helpless" (Reynolds 2006, x). He also makes it clear, though he says the discovery was "serendipitous" (Reynolds 2006, xi), that on more than one occasion he has used cooking as a means of seduction, to assert masculine sexual prowess, though he claims that the opposite (a woman cooking for a man) backfires because it gives the perception that the woman is needy. Despite one anecdote about how his strategy failed when he cooked an elaborate dinner for a woman and then she left at 10:00 pm to go on a second date, he claims that whereas taking a woman to a restaurant offers limited possibilities for showing off, "wielding a cleaver and sauté-ing diver scallops in [a man's] own kitchen, well, the work speaks for itself" (Reynolds 2006, xii). He even, somewhat tongue in cheek, offers his "Ten Rules for Seducing a Woman by Cooking Her Dinner" (Reynolds 2006, xiii). On the one hand, this has a bit of the feel of an outdated *Esquire* or *Playboy* piece; on the other hand, Reynolds is rather quick to laugh at his own sometimes-failed attempts as a kitchen Casanova.

As we see Reynolds continue to use food to shore up his feelings about masculinity, his narrative of how he manipulated his skills as a cook to help overcome disappointments in his career and personal life is both funny and disturbing. He aptly characterizes how preparing food became, on the one hand, a way of coping with personal disappointment, yet its ephemeral nature always left him wanting more:

> I began cooking to ward off uncertainty and depression, and it worked. But one of the drawbacks of cooking is also one of its joys—as creative works go, it's done quickly . . . and it's over quickly. Palliated as I was when planning and executing dinner for others (and even for myself), there was always a junkie's letdown the following day, when the eu-phoria evaporated and there was nothing tangible to show for it except garbage bags. (Reynolds 2006, 139)

Reynolds' culminating experience is a literal acting-out of the role that cooking has played in his life; in his play *Dinner with Demons* he prepares actual dishes (a deep-fried turkey, tomato sorbet, a potato soufflé, a giant apple pancake that he flips for the audience) on stage while talking about the events in his life to which each is connected—in the case of the apple pancake, for instance, he tells about eating it at a place called Reuben's when, as a junior in college, his mother threw him out of the house on Christmas Day for growing a beard. The performance itself represents an oddly purgatory-like repetition in which Reynolds must relive the events of his life (and must get the challenging act of cooking the food correctly before a live audience in real time) night after night; at the same time, he seems to use the performances as a way of mastering these events by turning them into drama. It is striking that when he talks about the "voice inside my head" that he can never get rid of during the performances (Reynolds 2006, 313), it is not a self-reflective or critical voice but rather one that worries about what the audience is thinking.

In an even more directed way, Bob Spitz in *The Saucier's Apprentice* (2008) sends himself on a journey through the cooking schools of Europe when his marriage ends badly and he feels conflicted about his current relation-ship: this may sound suspiciously like Elizabeth Gilbert's *Eat, Pray, Love*, but Spitz's obsessive emphasis on cooking techniques and his disarming honesty about his difficulty in dealing with the others in his classes makes this work introspective and nuanced. The memoir begins and ends with two dinner parties. At the first, Spitz lets us see how neurotically and obsessively—but how badly—he executes an overambitious menu for his friends. Recently divorced and having just completed an eight-year book project, he is at loose ends and freely admits that he is carrying a large burden of anger around with him: "For several months, I'd been storming around in a cloud of rage, like a bee-stung character in one of those Warner Brothers cartoons" (Spitz 2008, 14). Cooking for him, at least at first, is an outlet for that rage: "I took refuge in the kitchen. Somehow, amid the knives and icepicks, I felt safe there . . . There was nothing a bedraggled and broke, ex-metropolitan, middle-aged, divorced, pussy-whipped writer couldn't pull off in the kitchen if he followed directions" (Spitz 2008, 15).

Undertaking a European odyssey in order to find calm and direction through cooking is a venture Spitz both pokes fun at and justifies as not atypical of the middle-aged male's effort at self-discovery:

> Guys I know pursue countless flaky obsessions—a single-engine Cessna, a kitschy tattoo, that twenty-four-year-old trophy wife. Many of us today have the luxury and disposable income to pursue fantasies in ways our fathers never could. Somehow, with everything else falling apart around me, the one passion I was still sure of was cooking. (Spitz 2008, 32)

More self-aware as a memoirist than he seems to have been at the time of his experiences, Spitz lets us understand the difference between his infatuation with his then-girlfriend, Carolyn, and her ambivalence (or even disdain) for him. When she predictably dumps him after promising to join him on his cooking trip, he—like Gilbert—continues the trip as an effort toward some kind of enlightenment. Oddly enough, his first cooking teacher in France, Robert Ash, is both mentor and double. Like Spitz, he is an ex rock and roller, and each day of cooking ends in a raucous guitar jam session. At the same time, he insists on a level of perfectionism as a chef that proves to be a revelation to Spitz, who had always rushed pell-mell through his cooking preparations.

Most of the memoir, though, does not contain such magical meetings of mind. Spitz has a truly misanthropic side and is not afraid to let the reader see the extent to which his frustrations over his own behavior project themselves onto his feelings about others. Early on in his trip, Spitz is nearly seduced by a woman named Olivia, and then sees her in the café going through the same ritual with another man. Newly single, he is uncomfortable about the games one plays with the opposite sex, and seems to reserve a contempt bordering on misogyny for the occasional bimbos he encounters in the cooking classes on his journey, notably a young housewife named Didi and later a southern belle named Cheryl Lynn. While unwilling ever to show his true anger at having been jilted by Carolyn, he seems to take out these feelings on the various females he encounters during his trip. The one exception to this is Kate, one of his cooking teachers; his hyperawareness of her aloofness and her melancholy side makes her, like Robert Ash, one of the doppelganger figures with whom Spitz identifies: "there was something about Kate, a shadow within her . . . Perhaps it was the alienation, the price of living alone . . . Perhaps it was too close to issues I was wrangling with" (Spitz 2008, 162).

What makes Spitz's memoir remarkable as a whole is that his journey is almost a deromanticization of the cooking school experience; not only is he often critical of his fellow participants, but even some of his teacher-chefs, such as the mysterious Madame or the disorganized Frederic Riviere, also don't escape his unflattering depictions of their pedagogy (or lack thereof). Yet he stops just short of becoming holier-than-thou and actually opens a space within himself to appreciate people who lack his own culinary expertise. Late in the memoir, when he meets two husbands named Todd and Scott who are just learning to cook, he is initially contemptuous of them, but something changes in his attitude and he registers the pleasure of their excitement as novices: "It was like encountering two junkies. They had the same steamy energy about them, working off a food high, and I stood off to one side, envious of their discovery" (Spitz 2008, 252). The dinner party that ends the memoir shows how Spitz has indeed changed. He describes the elaborate preparations he makes, now informed by the poise, skills, and timing he has acquired on his trip: but the surprise ending is that he is not making the food to impress colleagues or his new girlfriend, but instead, the entire meal is solely for his young daughter, Lily. While Gilbert's memoir ends with her finding love (or at least sex) with her Brazilian in Bali, Spitz's redemptive force lies in the return home, the embracing of his maternal side, and the acceptance of own difficulties with his masculine roles.

Frank Bruni's *Born Round* (2009) takes an entirely different perspective. Bruni spent years as the restaurant critic for the *New York Times*, but what we learn in the memoir is that this prestigious position only came after a lifetime of experiencing a deeply ambivalent relationship with food and with his own body image, a concern that one normally sees in parallel works by women writers. Bruni begins the memoir with the offer of the food critic position for the *New York Times*, then uses the moment to flash back to the love/hate relationship he has held with food since childhood. He explains, "My life-defining relationship, after all, wasn't with a parent, a sibling, a teacher, a mate. It was with my stomach" (Bruni 2009, 5). If this sounds like a surprising revelation for a man, it is even more surprising to learn in the early portions of the memoir that Bruni suffered from bulimia, an eating disorder more commonly associated with females, and that in his twenties he tried everything from speed to Prozac to grueling marathon runs in the effort to lose weight—and yet was so helpless against his tendency to binge that he would turn down dates or resort to strategies like keeping his windbreaker on the entire evening. Being an overweight gay man in a subculture obsessed with idealized, muscular male bodies did nothing to help his self-image.

In his early thirties, Bruni was assigned by the *Times* to cover Congress, and was shocked when he saw a photograph of himself: "Something strange happens when you keep gaining weight that you don't want to be gaining and keep breaking your resolutions to lose it: a part of your brain—the part that keeps your disappointment in yourself at a manageable level, trading real self-disgust for more routine self-flagellation—shades the truth a little and then a little more, and then a lot" (Bruni 2009, 203–4). While we have seen Reynolds and Spitz turn to cooking for others as a form of self-comfort, for Bruni, that effort manifests itself in the pure act of eating: "I ate to steady my nerves, to distract myself from my apprehension, to dull my occasional loneliness, to quell my sporadic boredom. I ate because I didn't have any dates on the next week's calendar or any romantic prospects in my sights and could postpone a new diet and a new discipline by a day, a week" (Bruni 2009, 205). There is both humor and recognition in the realization that as long as he is overweight, he can use it as an excuse for the other shortcomings in his life: "Being fat absolved me, in a sense, of so many other flaws. It took the blame for a whole host of setbacks and disappointments" (Bruni 2009, 207).

The problem reaches its crisis point just at a potential high for Bruni's journalism career when he becomes part of the press corps for the Bush campaign in January 2000. In part as an effort to keep the reporters from complaining, they are fed six or seven huge meals a day, and Bruni's blow-by-blow account of these feedings shows what he was up against. Only later, when he is reassigned to Rome, does he realize that though the Italians love food, it is the *way* they eat—small helpings, fine food, spread out over many hours—that constitutes for him a "reeducation" (Bruni 2009, 258). Shortly after this, he accepts the *Times* food critic position, but the demand that he try everything is still a constant struggle; at first, he even continues a secret commute back to Washington D.C. to work with his trainer.

Ironically, though, he realizes that through the sheer variety of what he has to eat, he can let go of the fear of not having enough that has always underscored his cravings: "Forced to eat a certain amount, I developed an ability not to eat too much more than that . . . And I had the challenge and diversion of coming to conclusions about everything I tried" (Bruni 2009, 326). Oddly enough, his work as a restaurant reviewer forces him to structure his eating in a more controlled way: rather than dieting, he says, "The structure I had now was based on indulgence, on what I *must* have, and that made all the difference. I was celebrating instead of abusing food" (Bruni 2009, 340). Of course, few others would have Bruni's singular opportunity to relearn one's eating habits by suddenly being given a huge expense account and being forced to eat multiple courses at high-end restaurants every night.

But Bruni's larger point is that by learning to let go of associating food with "guilt and shame" (Bruni 2009, 341), he was finally able to keep his binging in check, at least most of the time. Most important, he says, he had to learn not to lie to himself about food. Bruni's account of the problems he had accepting his own sexuality and his efforts at food-related self-denial provides a moving example of how the male food memoirist—by going public with such confessions—can give us a larger picture of how "wrestling with gravy" is indeed a male anxiety and a male creative source.

Marcus Samuelsson's *Yes, Chef* (2012) is different from these other memoirs insofar as Samuelsson's tricultural identity (he was adopted from Ethiopia, raised in Sweden, and now identifies with Harlem/New York City) plays a significant role. It is also necessary to point out that his memoir is "as told to" a distinguished writer in her own right, Veronica Chambers, but I feel that the voice and the experiences of the book are authentically Samuelsson's own, and also that its emphasis on identity as formed through food—and later redefined as part of yet another "male midlife crisis" narrative—links it to the other works that I have discussed in this chapter.

Samuelsson's very earliest memories are of his mother in Ethiopia, though he says he has never seen a picture of her and doesn't remember her voice. She died of tuberculosis shortly after bringing Marcus and his sister to a hospital; a Swedish couple adopted the two children from an orphanage in Ethiopia in 1972. His upbringing, then, was a Swedish one, complete with fishing trips and the traditional cuisine of that country. He says that his love of food did not come from his adoptive mother, who had very little time to cook and who kept a rigid weekly menu schedule, though it was from his mother that he learned how to persuade the fishmonger to give them the freshest fish. The significant culinary presence in his childhood was his adoptive grandmother, Mormor, who taught him how to prepare a traditional roast chicken with spices. Also significant for Marcus was a fishing trip he took as a child with his father and uncle; he was entrusted to prepare the dinner for them, which he did with great care, and so it was within this kind of fatherly/masculine space that he experienced his first sense of triumph as a cook.

As a young Black man in Sweden, where there were very few others who looked like him, Samuelsson encountered his share of racism as a child, which also shaped his later feelings about his identity. He recalls verbal abuse on the playground as a child, and being turned down for a job at McDonald's due to probable bigotry. As he became an avid soccer player, though, it was striking to him that his teammates—even the white ones—referred to themselves as *Blatte*, "a historically derogatory term for immigrants that my generation claimed with pride" (Samuelsson 2012, 43). When he was turned down for the chance to play soccer professionally, though, he entered a vocational high school and began his serious training as a chef. The cook's knife that his parents gave him for his seventeenth birthday marked an acknowledgement of his choice and a masculine rite of passage.

In the middle parts of the memoir, we see his struggle to distinguish himself within a very rigid and autocratic restaurant training system. When he goes to Switzerland to train under Herr Stocker, a notoriously demanding chef, his anxiety is so great that he experiences daily nausea and vomiting (while Bruni's vomiting was self-induced, it connects to Samuelsson's experience in the sense that both men paradoxically loved food, yet manifested their fears through the rejection of it). The other point of crisis for Samuelsson in this part of the narrative occurs when he impregnates a girlfriend, Brigitta, and his parents end up insisting that he/they send support money to the daughter that she has as a result, though he does not actually meet her until many years later. He also still must contend with the casual racism of the culinary world in, for example, the way that his boss uses the term "nègres" to refer to the "underlings" in the kitchen. After a pleasure trip on which he loses his closest friend in a car accident, though, in his grief he seeks another restaurant placement, and ends up immigrating to New York City.

In New York for the first time, he is struck by the fact that he is surrounded by others who look like him: when he lands at JFK, "the first thing I noticed were all the black people" (Samuelsson 2012, 134). And yet, having grown up in Sweden, he knows next to nothing about African American culture—about the history of the Civil Rights movement, about rap music, about soul food, and so forth. He begins work at Aquavit, a Swedish fine-dining restaurant, and is highly successful at his craft. By playing soccer for recreation, he is able to make friends who are, like him, both Black and Swedish. Yet he still feels marginalized as a Black man who is a professional chef; he says that at this time, with the exception of Patrick Clark, "black people were almost by design not part of the conversation about fine dining" (Samuelsson 2012, 151). Determined to internationalize his palate, he takes a job as a chef on a cruise ship, where he is not permitted to be particularly creative but where he learns from his Filipino crewmates, tries different foods at every port, and writes avidly in his food journal. In order to achieve the highest level of credentials as a chef, he finally gets his longed-for position training in France under Georges Blanc.

During the period of Samuelsson's training in France and his subsequent return to helm the kitchen at Aquavit (where, under his direction as head chef, the restaurant receives a coveted three star review from the *New York Times*), he finds himself having to suppress almost every aspect of the feelings generated from events that happen in his personal life: his grief over his grandmother's death; his daughter, Zoe, whom none of his colleagues know about; and his sense of being "rudderless" (Samuelsson 2012, 201) after his father dies but he can't, because of his immigration status, attend the funeral. His longing to be able to express familial connections plays a key role in what will soon become his moment of crisis action.

The other key set of events that helps to precipitate his crisis action concerns his growing frustration with the racism in the chef world. He recounts, for instance, a scenario in which celebrity chef Gordon Ramsay, angry that Samuelsson doesn't mention his name when he comes to London and reporters interview him, calls him a "fucking black bastard" (Samuelsson 2012, 211). He points out that although in some ways the restaurant industry is known for its tolerance (of gay people and of immigrants, for example), "blacks, and especially American blacks, are shamefully underrepresented at the high end of the business" (Samuelsson 2012, 213), and he goes on to list five different theories about "why kitchens remain so white" (Samuelsson 2012, 213). This question of racial identity leads Samuelsson to begin to form more of a consciousness that is an activist one as well as an introspective one; he says that although he was initially uncomfortable dealing with race as a way that people saw him, "the more I traveled around the country, the more I came to see my race as an opportunity rather than a burden" (Samuelsson 2012, 215). The turning point comes, though, when he is speaking at the French Culinary Institute and a young black student asks him a question about the current cooking trends in Africa. He realizes at this moment that he has no idea how to answer: "I felt as if I'd been slapped into awareness. I felt unsettled. Why *didn't* I know more about African food? Why was I so clueless about Ethiopian cuisine, when it was the country of my birth?" (Samuelsson 2012, 217).

It is at this point that Samuelsson embarks upon some major changes in his life, one of which involves the first of several journeys back to Ethiopia not simply to learn more about its food culture, but more important, to find a connection to his lost biological family members there. He remarks that during his first two weeks there, "I saw my own face reflected a thousand times over, which not only gave me a sense of belonging unlike I'd had anywhere else in my life, but also a deep reminder of how fate had steered my life on such a different course" (Samuelsson 2012, 222). On a later trip, he even gets the opportunity to meet Tsegie, his birth father, and ends up supporting the opportunity for his young half-sisters to attend school, despite their father's initial resistance.

The next major step he takes, emboldened by having met these biological family members, is to reconnect with Zoe, the daughter that he had with Brigitta, who was now a teenager. When he goes to see her in Austria, he uses cooking—potato-apple soup and chocolate blinis—as a way to overcome the awkwardness and forge a connection with her. "Each night in Austria," he says, "I cooked a meal that I hoped would bring me a little closer to winning Zoe over. I was reaching out the only way I knew how. I cooked her the dishes of my childhood" (Samuelsson 2012, 257). Although he finds the experience emotionally overwhelming, and has to deal later, when Zoe comes to visit him in New York, with her "feelings of betrayal and loss" (Samuelsson 2012, 259) over his having been absent from her life for so many years, he admits to his satisfaction with the idea of working on re-forming the relationship. It is also around this time that he marries his girlfriend, Maya, with a traditional wedding back in Ethiopia.

Samuelsson's life-altering decision to make a connection to his family in Ethiopia also ends up sending his cooking passions even further away from traditional Swedish cuisine and more in the direction of African and African-American cuisine. He opens a pan-African restaurant, Merkato, but it fails due to problematic business partners. At the same time that he is becoming involved in mentoring young Black chefs, he engages in a legal battle in which he literally has to buy back the rights to his own name in order to use it independently in his career outside of Aquavit. This marks another crisis in his identity, as he considers going back to his Ethiopian birth name, Kassahun Tsegie, but ultimately has to pay the money to his ex-business partner in order to retain the name by which people recognize him. Poignantly, he remarks that he would have changed his name in a heartbeat years ago if it had meant the chance for a green card:

> But what I know now that I didn't know then is that our names are our stories. We sew our experiences together to make a life and our names are both the needle and the thread. "Marcus Samuelsson" is more than the name of a chef who has done X, Y, and Z. It's a name that reflects my life: where I started, each stop along my journey, and the man that I've become. (Samuelsson 2012, 279)

By the end of the memoir, Samuelsson has reached a pinnacle in his career by competing on and winning Top Chef Masters and by being chosen to cook President Obama's first state dinner. Even more important in terms of his identity, though, is that although he is African rather than African American by birth, he has become deeply attached to the history and culture of Harlem, and opens a restaurant there, Red Rooster, that he (at least in theory, since it quickly became a celebrity hot spot) envisioned as a neighborhood anchor for creative, internationally influenced soul food and a desirable place of employment for African American food workers. He says, "If I kept my heart in the right place and steeped myself in Harlem's history, then the people would come— and keep coming" (Samuelsson 2012, 298). He adds that he sees Harlem as "diverse enough . . . to encompass" everything that he is: "After all that traveling, I am, at last, home" (Samuelsson 2012, 315). Like Reynolds and Spitz, he is driven by a sense of loss, of being untethered, and it is through the meeting of food and geography that he finds a kind of rootedness (as we will also see in the writers discussed in the next chapter); just as he himself was adopted, he adopts a new cultural history. And like Bourdain and Bruni, as he becomes famous, he has difficulty knowing where his public persona stops and his "real" self begins—but always, he realizes that cooking allows him to create his own kind of truth.

EIGHT

School Lunch

Bicultural Conflicts in Asian-American Women's Food Memoirs

To write as a successful chef or food critic is, of course, to write from a place of privilege. The acknowledgment of one's eating practices as a conscious choice underscores the difference that Deane W. Curtin delineates between those who are preoccupied with food because they choose to be, and those who do so because they have to (Curtin 1992, 4). This chapter returns to the question of the need—the hunger—that is fulfilled by an attempt to make sense of one's food experiences as inflected by such factors as social class, religion, race or ethnicity, and of course one's gender. Among the recent wave of food memoirs by women writers, some of the standout works have dealt specifically with the experience of bicultural and/or immigrant identity. These include Diana Abu-Jaber's *The Language of Baklava* (discussed in chapter 6) about growing up in upstate New York in a Jordanian-American family; Kim Sunée's *Trail of Crumbs* (also discussed in chapter 6) about being adopted from Korea, growing up in New Orleans, and seeking an adult identity in Provence; and Shoba Narayan's *Monsoon Diary*, about being raised in India and facing culture shock upon attending college in the United States. Nowhere is it more apparent, though, what kinds of struggles these writers undergo as children than in the arena of the school lunchroom—a site that even many of us who are non-immigrants will remember as highly contested. For the mother or grandmother who prepares traditional dishes, the loving desire to pass these foods on to the daughter or granddaughter is a strongly marked cultural imperative. But for the daughter or granddaughter under pressure to assimilate into an American venue—

particularly one as fraught with competition and bigotry as the lunch-room—not having the "right" foods seems to spell trouble. While this issue obviously applies to immigrant kids from many different back-grounds, my focus on the school lunch battle in this chapter is primarily on food memoirs by Asian-American women writers: Bich Minh Nguy-en's *Stealing Buddha's Dinner* and Linda Furiya's *Bento Box in the Heart-land*. Both of these works play out the bicultural Asian-American daugh-ter's subjectivity issues through the daily problem of school lunch. As a kind of counternarrative, I will conclude with a brief look at Ava Chin's recent memoir, *Eating Wildly*. In a certain sense, Chin's book rewrites the anxieties over food identities by using foraging as an alternative ap-proach that rejects the bilateral "choices" of immigrant or American cul-tural values in favor of forms of improvisation.

Stealing Buddha's Dinner is Nguyen's memoir of her girlhood as part of a family of refugees from Viet Nam who ended up in Grand Rapids, Michigan. Throughout the work, Bich finds herself torn between her tra-ditional Vietnamese grandmother, Noi (her missing mother is a signifi-cant theme in the book), and an obsessively frugal Chicana stepmother, Rosa; her school lunch, for economic as well as cultural reasons, can never live up to the Betty Crockerlike perfection of the other girls whom she so deeply envies.

School lunch plays a dominant role in Bich's longings for assimilation. During the periods of her school years when she and her siblings go home for lunch, Noi makes traditional Vietnamese dishes such as steam-ing bowls of shrimp *mi* soup and seared steaks (Nguyen 2007, 83). At home, Bich is free to embrace the deliciousness of Noi's cooking, her *pho*, the fragrant and spicy beef soup with noodles. But when she must bring lunch to school, it is another story altogether. At her elementary school, as is the case for most of us who have ever had to bring a packed lunch to school, "a student was measured by the contents of her lunch bag, which displayed status, class, and parental love" (Nguyen 2007, 75). It is not Noi's dishes that raise the conflicts here, but rather, Bich's stepmother Rosa's refusal to emulate what Bich sees as certain lunchroom impera-tives. Bich detests the cheap lunchmeat that Rosa buys, the generic cook-ies: "Rosa bought whatever white bread was cheapest—sadly, never the Wonder Bread my friends ate, which I was certain had a fluffier, more luxurious bite—and peanut butter and jelly, olive loaf, or thin packets of pastrami and corned beef made by a company called Buddig" (Nguyen 2007, 76). In Bich's mind, Rosa's frugality is a key contributor to her own inability to fit in with her peers, as she pictures herself having a different life if she were mothered into the mainstream. She longs to have what she considers a "real" mother like her friend Holly does: "No one cared more than Holly Jansen's mom" (Nguyen 2007, 78).

Holly's lunches, with her thermos of Campbell's chicken-noodle soup and her Tupperware containers, make Bich almost sick with envy: "I watched as Holly unlatched the Tupperware and drew from it her first course: a sandwich wrapped like a gift in wax paper. Holly's sandwiches were never limp or squashed, battered by books in a schoolbag" (Nguyen 2007, 79). This is followed by a paragraph that defines Holly's sandwiches and the rest of her lunch in terms of what it is not (i.e., the ways that it fails to resemble Bich's own). Bich's subjectivity—which for her as a child is defined through food—is described perpetually in terms of loss, envy, and failure. She takes a secret pleasure in reading the items on the hot lunch menu at school offered for lower-income kids, but cannot admit any desire to partake in it and therefore to sink even lower on the status ladder: "The implicit judgment was that if you had to get lunch from the cafeteria, your mom didn't care enough" (Nguyen 2007, 78). What is at work here as well is the notable absence of Bich's mother from most of the memoir: her mother was separated from the rest of the family when they immigrated to the United States, and so Bich's feelings of anger and of envy of other people's families are complicated by her own feelings of lack. When she finally is invited to Holly's house for a sleepover, Bich is mortified when she unintentionally commits several breaches of etiquette, including not knowing to say grace or put her napkin on her lap, and feeling lost when Holly's mother serves pork chops and she has no idea how to cut them with a fork and knife. She admits to herself that the pork chops themselves are horribly overcooked and not nearly as delicious as Noi's *pho*, "[b]ut the lesson hard-learned at Holly's stayed with me" (Nguyen 2007, 93). Determinedly, Bich begins to eat all of her meals with a knife and fork—both Holly's family's way, and the European way, which Rosa shows her—from then on. Later breaches of etiquette happen when, for instance, Bich eats dinner at her friend Tara's house and unknowingly sits at the head of the table, the father's place: "I hadn't yet learned the rules about fathers and mothers, head and foot, the king and his castle" (Nguyen 2007, 119).

Bich's longing for American food, especially candy and junk food, represents the almost transubstantive feeling that by consuming the embodiments of American culture, she will somehow become more American. Her fascination with Pringles, with the way that Pringles come stacked so neatly in a can, is a telling example: "Anh [her sister] and I were transfixed by the bright red cylinder and the mustachioed grin on Mr. Pringles's broad, pale face" (Nguyen 2007, 3). And in another moment, her list of favored types of candy reads like a kind of poetry (Nguyen 2007, 50–51). (In fact, when my Literature of Food class conducted a conference call interview with Bich after studying the book, her voice still became dreamy and nostalgic when one of my students asked her whether she still liked the same candies.) Nestle's Toll House cookies, for her, become a metonymic representation of both her longing and her feelings of rejection: "each chocolate chip cookie [was] a reminder of the toll, the price of admission into a long-desired house" (Nguyen 2007, 71).

It is clear throughout the memoir that there is an extent to which Bich, in her innermost self, remains loyal to her family's Vietnamese traditions; her favorite part of the evening is when Noi slices fruit and shares it with the Buddha in her room and with Bich and her sister: "The presentation meant a winding-down into bedtime and made me feel warm, safe" (Nguyen 2007, 29). Yet when her school has a version of a Tet celebration and Noi donates a plate full of *banh chung* (green sticky rice cakes), the two sisters sneak most of the plate's contents for themselves, reasoning that it will be subject to ridicule or rejection by their classmates: "we knew then they [the rice cakes] would be going to the Land of Sharing, of white people looking and declining. The cakes would grow crusty and stale under the recoiling gazes of our classmates. They would be ruined by the staring" (Nguyen 2007, 102). Bich's outward gaze is toward the labels and packages of the American junk foods she covets; it is a desire to appropriate by looking and by consuming. The reversal of that gaze, though, is a judgment, a rejection, an affirmation of otherness. The cakes themselves are depicted as "ruined by the staring," as if the imperialist gaze has a destructive power all its own. Bich's ambivalence comes in her desire to protect the cakes, or to consume them for herself, but her anger that the power to "ruin" comes from the very place into which she longs to assimilate. In a sense, the memoir as a whole acts out this ambivalence; as an adult narrator, Bich can reflect on the immense power that American consumer ideals held over her, but she can convey the price she has paid in her feelings of loss, longing, and marginalization.

Linda Furiya's *Bento Box in the Heartland*, like *Stealing Buddha's Dinner*, uses the fish-out-of-water motif of a childhood in an immigrant family not in an urban setting like Los Angeles or New York City, but again, in the American heartland. Furiya's father was born in California but raised by his grandfather in Japan and was not able to return to the United States for many years because he was stripped of his citizenship during World War II and later spent three years in a Russian POW camp; when his American citizenship was reinstated, he got work in the Midwest as a chick sexer and chose his Japanese wife, who came to the United States to marry him, through a matchmaker. Linda's family is even more isolated than Bich's, as her parents have settled in Versailles, a rural Indiana community near the Ohio border, and have almost no other Asian families around them. Her father plants a garden for her mother and attempts to grow the vegetables and herbs that she wants, but trips to the Asian markets in big cities like Cincinnati and Chicago are rare and significant.

At school, the other children blur her identity into an undifferentiated anti-Asian bigotry, making fun of her slanted eyes and calling her a "Chink" or a "Jap" (Furiya 2006, 7)—until she learns to fight back by calling them vicious names in return. More so than in Nguyen's memoir, Linda feels keenly the difference in English skills between herself and her parents. She recounts her embarrassment when store clerks fail to under-stand her father's accent, erupting in anger on his behalf at the meat counter: "'What is your problem?' I yelled, waving my hands, 'Don't you understand English? Won't you just *try* to *listen* to what he's saying?'" (Furiya 2006, 210). But she stops at the acknowledgment that her efforts to make the clerk recognize her frustration are futile. Her mother, a stay-at-home mom who attempts to teach herself English by watching soap operas, is less fluent than her father and relies upon Linda from a very young age, to do things like make phone calls to repairmen and write school attendance notes: "As an American-born child, writing letters and making phone calls wasn't a difficult task, but knowing my mother couldn't do it, or was afraid to, and that she depended on me made it a weighty responsibility" (Furiya 2006, 207). Although Linda focuses pri-marily on her childhood in her memoir, her occasional flashes forward show her attempts to explore the differences between her anger at her mother at the time, and her later feelings of empathy: abruptly, for in-stance, at one moment she says, "When I lived in China with my baby boy, I came to understand the isolation my mother faced in raising a family in a small town in Indiana" (Furiya 2006, 41).

And like Bich, Linda loves the traditional foods that her family eats for lunch at home. When her mother is not packing a bento box for her father to bring to work, they have what Linda describes as "magnificent feasts" for lunch: appetizers of "spicy wilted cabbage" with lemon peel, chili peppers, garlic, and kombu; "cubes of tofu garnished with ginger and bonito flakes"; grilled salmon or steak with onions, soy sauce, and rice wine; miso soup, and rice (Furiya 2006, 4). However, once at school, she learns very quickly that this must be kept a secret if she is to hope for any acceptance by her peers: "My very first notion of how different we really were struck me among the pastel-colored molded trays and long bleached wood tables of the school cafeteria" (Furiya 2006, 3). At first, Linda assumes that when she opens the lunch her mother has packed for her, it will resemble the other kids': "My stomach lurched. I expected a classic elementary school lunch of a bologna, cheese, and Miracle Whip sandwich and a bag of Durkee's potato sticks, but all I saw were three round rice balls wrapped in waxed paper. Mom had made me an *obento*, a Japanese-style boxed meal" (Furiya 2006, 5).

Her recourse becomes a kind of dual duplicity, both to her classmates and to her mother. To her classmates, Linda pretends steadily that all she has for lunch is an apple and a cookie; she actually prefers the idea that "[t]he lunch box crowd voted unanimously that my mother packed the lamest lunches in history" (Furiya 2006, 11) to letting them see the *onigiri*, or rice balls, that her lunch box contains. But since her mother knows how much she actually loves the *onigiri*, Linda has to give up on request-ing that her mother pack her a sandwich. Rather, she develops a secret binging ritual of consuming them in a stall in the girls' bathroom, thus pleasing her mother by bringing home an empty lunch box. Her description of the *onigiri* shows her actual pleasure in their taste and texture: "the crunchy seaweed wrapping . . . the salty rice . . . the surprise center, a buttery chunk of salmon," with "centers of pickled plum and silky kelp" in the others (Furiya 2006, 10). Interestingly, rather than resenting the perceived need to consume the *onigiri* secretly in the bathroom, she experiences it as an act of empowerment (somewhat akin to the ways that bulimics, as in former *New York Times* restaurant critic Frank Bruni's *Born Round*, may view their clandestine purging rituals). Furiya writes, "It was a secret act that I found empowering and primal, rather than diminishing. I was hungry, and yet there was an odd sense of invincibility, the banishment of fear . . . I had the sensation that if I left one grain uneaten, something inside me would shrivel up and die. I took big mouthfuls of the rice and chewed as fast as I could until there was no more" (Furiya 2006, 10).

Like Bich, Linda has a sleepover story, but with a different setting and outcome. Aware of the extreme differences between her own household and that of her friend Tracy (as Bich does, she describes the family sitting quietly at the dinner table with their napkins on their laps), Linda is unwilling to invite white school friends to spend the night at her own house: "The differences reflected at my home were glaring. We had to take our shoes off at the door. My parents spoke a foreign language. In our kitchen, a wok was poised on the burner instead of a cast-iron skillet . . . A bottle of soy sauce and a shaker of *togarashi* (mixed red peppers) were coupled with peanut butter and strawberry preserves. I wanted to keep these details within the walls of my house" (Furiya 2006, 69). Contrary to her expectations—and contrary to Bich's experiences with her neighbor Jennifer, who rejects all food offered by Noi—Tracy is enthralled by the origami cranes that Linda's mother makes, by the Japanese omelet with *tonkatsu* sauce, and by the mother's stories about the past. This marks a turning point in Linda's willingness to take an interest in her own parents' backgrounds, but she is also "left with a gnawing insecurity and jealousy" (Furiya 2006, 79). She finds old family photo albums, including a shot taken of her mother as she boarded the plane to go to America to meet her new husband for the first time, but she is afraid to ask questions. Throughout the memoir, we see the young Linda's curiosity about the past mixed with the fear that to veer in that direction is to find out things she is afraid to know; Bich's unwillingness to ask questions about her absent mother reflects a similar set of fears. Interestingly, Linda's father—unlike her mother—seems far more willing to talk about his own difficult past, but only while the family is eating: "For Dad, it was always food—the setting of a meal or its sensual characteristics—that struck a chord of nostalgia" (Furiya 2006, 46). Bich's family attempts at various intervals to bond over shared meals at American chains like Ponderosa, but there is never a sense that communal reflection about the past is encouraged or desired, and the food itself—the Ponderosa buffet that seemed at first to be sumptuous—gradually loses its appeal.

Later in *Bento Box*, when a Vietnamese immigrant girl, Tam, arrives, the local families assume that they will become instant friends: "I thought you would all be like distant cousins or something," says Mrs. Anders (Furiya 2006, 184). But as it becomes clear that she and her family are even less assmiliated and speak even less English, Linda feels deeply resentful and rebuffs Tam's attempts at friendship. While Bich sees Holly as the other whom she longs to be, Tam is the other self that Linda hates and fears: "It took me a long time to admit to myself that it was because I was ashamed, and that I disliked Tam because she wasn't Americanized enough for me. She made me remember the insecure girl who saw her true Asian reflection in the store window at the mall" (Furiya 2006, 193).

Both memoirs end, as is frequently the case in the immigrant memoir genre, with the narrator achieving a kind of reconciliation with the past by means of a return visit to the homeland. Bich, as an adult, journeys to Vietnam with Noi and meets her extended family for the first time since infancy; Linda, as a teenager, goes to Japan with her mother and learns more about the aspects of her culture that she had previously viewed with ambivalence. (And in her sequel, *How to Cook a Dragon*, she spends part of her young adult life in China, where she deals with even more complicated versions of ethnic confusion, but learns to embrace the language and the cuisine.) However, I want to close this part of my discussion by noting a key difference in narrative technique between Nguyen's work and Furiya's work that reflects their choices in what we might call "food memoir language." As I discussed in the introduction to this volume, one fascinating aspect of the food memoir is the authors' decisions about whether to incorporate recipes into the text of the narrative. Again, some authors whose preoccupation is an ambivalent relationship between their present and the food of the past do not include recipes; *Born Round* by Frank Bruni (discussed in the previous chapter) falls into this category, as does *Stealing Buddha's Dinner*. Furiya, on the other hand, uses a recipe from her mother to end each chapter of the book, a technique we see in many other food memoirs, though sometimes used more playfully, as in Abu-Jaber's *The Language of Baklava*. To offer a recipe for a traditional dish is an acknowledgment of both a debt and a continuation. Yet it is also a form of re-appropriation, for the author has always taken its language, its narrative, and even the way it is presented and served—these ingredients of the past—and made them her own.

Ava Chin's *Eating Wildly: Foraging for Life, Love, and the Perfect Meal* is both a part of the genre of food memoirs by Asian-American women, and a book that takes an entirely different approach to the question of how to come to terms with one's cultural past and present identity as expressed through cooking and eating. Chin, who was largely raised by her grandparents in Flushing, Queens (her father was absent and her mother was busy dating), expresses longing and reverence for the kinds of traditional Chinese foods that her grandparents prepared for her. She says that her grandfather, "a former Toisanese village boy turned Chinese restaurant worker, taught me how to eat" (Chin 2014, 12) and adds, "By four years old, I was already cracking open crabs with a nutcracker and devouring lobsters from claw to tail" (Chin 2014, 13). The memoir is filled with vivid, nostalgic depictions of the dishes that her grandparents made, but as the grandfather and then later the grandmother dies, it also becomes a story of loss and longing. Unlike Nguyen and Furiya—and in part because she is a third rather than second-generation storyteller—Chin craves a deeper connection to the past rather than an assimilation into normative American eating practices.

As an adult, unmoored and facing grief, Chin creates a new way of understanding her past and present identity by training herself as a food forager. This allows her to redefine herself professionally (she begins to write the Urban Forager column for the *New York Times* and of course eventually this memoir itself), but far more significant than that is the way that foraging serves as a structuring metaphor for her own subjectivity. Foraging, which involves discovering and using otherwise-neglected ingredients such as the various mushrooms that grow in parks and even in the sidewalk cracks in New York City, connects her to her grandfather and her memory of accompanying him to Chinese grocers where he knew how to create magical dishes out of esoteric market finds. In the midst of the extreme grief that she feels while reflecting on her grandmother's bitterness toward her father, for instance, a wintertime discovery of reishi in Prospect Park (Brooklyn) gives her comfort:

> I sat there on that log, marveling at the resiliency of nature and the earth's ability to provide. Even among the coldest layer of frost there were plants and mushrooms that embraced winter, as well as other, more hidden things—roots, fungi, and seeds—all lying dormant, awaiting the arrival of spring. (Chin 2014, 51)

Foraging is both a literal and a figurative digging up of treasure, a reminder of what one already has as well as a promise of something new. But it also involves a kind of improvisation or *bricolage* in present-day life, which becomes a way of cherishing the unexpected and being the agent of one's own happiness. In the later parts of the memoir, Chin takes pleasure not only in finding a partner who is a fellow forager, but also in finally understanding how foraging has taught her a crucial level of self-reliance:

> In many ways, perhaps I was also the perfect person to become a forager. What had started with the search for my father was soon followed up by all those years yearning for a real love to fulfill me. It was only

until I started looking for my own food, getting to know the edible plants and mushrooms all around me, that I had started to understand that everything in nature was cyclical, everything interrelated. And the timing of things was key . . . Instead of wishing for something or someone to be there that wasn't, I could now see clearly before me what was. (Chin 2014, 224–25)

Like Furiya, Chin includes recipes throughout the memoir; here, though, since the recipes involve foraged ingredients, their narrative relation to the reader is complicated by our potential expertise—or more likely, lack of expertise—in finding them. Using foraged ingredients inherently makes a recipe riskier than, say, the potential for dough not to rise or for a cake to burn, since an incorrect choice can be poison: for example, in her recipe for Field Garlic and Hummus, Chin warns the reader who is searching for field garlic to "[b]eware of poisonous look-alikes" (Chin 2014, 35). The reader and cook, then, is invited actively to experience both the pleasure and the danger of foraging, an act of sharing embodied as well in the inclusion of dishes from foraged ingredients that Chin eventually prepares for family, friends, and even (in the volume's final recipe, when she enters a cooking contest) strangers. To forage is to take embodied creative risks, but it is also to share and to teach.

This trio of memoirists—Nguyen, Furiya, and Chin—illustrates the layers of narrative and emotional complexity involved in second and third generation immigrant food writing. All three of these women are to some extent the "angry daughters" portrayed in chapter 6, but more than that, Nguyen and Furiya depict the tremendous anger and ambivalence about their cultural identities caused by peer pressure and the longing for assimilation into normative American society; Chin's story, however, emphasizes the freedom that becomes available through the recognition of one's literal and figurative roots and through the desire to use them when concocting a new space and place for one's identity.

Conclusion

When we "read" a plate of food, we engage in much of the same activity that we do when we read a book. The initial presentation is, like the cover of a book, one we first take in visually, and make immediate judgments. Is it simple, or fancy? What does the material of the cover or plate look like? What images of status or class does it attempt to confer (with, on a plate of restaurant food for example, the use of drizzled sauces or the architectural layering of ingredients)? While the coinage "Instagrammable" might not often apply to book covers, it pops up again and again these days on cooking shows and in culinary magazines as a shorthand way of saying that some effort has been put into the initial appearance.

And taking the first bite is like reading the opening paragraph: our expectations are high, but does that initial taste of narrative or of food live up to its promise? And to what extent do our impressions reshape themselves as we proceed further in the act of reading or eating? Perhaps we become bored or satiated and push the book or plate aside. Or perhaps we go back for more. As the book comes to an end, we might hope for an epilogue, or a sequel, or we might comb the internet afterward for reviews so that we can see what others thought of it. At the end of the meal, we might throw the plate into the sink or dishwasher and get on with the day, or we might savor a dessert, a cup of coffee, or—if we are feeling especially decadent—an after-dinner liqueur. As this volume comes to a close, I offer three more small portions—a tasting plate of desserts, if you will—as final considerations of how the "literature of food" continues to be a vital, appetizing part of contemporary culture.

When Eric Schlosser wrote *Fast Food Nation* (parts of which originally appeared in *Rolling Stone* magazine) in 2001–2002, and Morgan Spurlock made his infamous documentary *Super Size Me* about the effect of eating McDonald's at every meal for a month, it marked a crucial moment of change in the way we read our plates: we were now asking questions such as how the chickens or cows were cared for before they came to us as food, how the workers were treated who created what we were eating, and what kinds of chemicals we were involuntarily ingesting. "McDonaldization" became a term and even the title of a series of articles (see Ritzer, 2002), while the disparities between starvation and obesity in America and other countries became increasingly marked (see Popkin, 2009). Novelist Jonathan Safran Foer (author of *Everything is Illuminated* and *Extremely Loud and Incredibly Close*) wrote an impassioned memoir about vegetarianism called *Eating Animals*. Mark Bittman and Michael Pollan, both extremely influential food writers, urged us to change our eating habits so that we were consuming less meat and eating more mindfully (more "real" or whole foods, fewer commercially processed ones): the mantra of Pollan's *In Defense of Food* was "Eat food. Not too much. Mostly plants" (Pollan 2008, 1).

While the works by Schlosser, Pollan, and others are not strictly literary (although director Richard Linklater did adapt *Fast Food Nation* into a feature film), they are nonetheless valuable in terms of how we consider food both in real life and in the narrative modes I have explored in the preceding pages. The real-life applications are obvious ones: many of us, as a result of their work, have become much more conscious and conscientious consumers. What I would suggest here, though, is that there is a clear analogy between what Schlosser, Pollan, et al. are doing and what close readers of literary food writing might do. Both involve an act of *mindfulness*, of paying close attention to materiality (again, as informed by OOOT), and of embracing rather than rejecting the physically present, acculturated body as part of the narrative.

We are reminded, too, that just as books are the product of the mental and physical labor of their authors (and editors, publishers, etc.), food comes to us through the labor of those who produce it, from the farmers to the purveyors to the cooks. This brings us to our second "after-dinner" offering: an attention to food as *work*. When we finish a meal at a restaurant, we may not give much thought to the busser who clears our dishes or to the minimum-wage worker who puts them into the dish machine, but they are of course present. One subgenre of the culinary memoir that I have not discussed in the previous chapters is that of the restaurant worker. Certainly, there have been popular food memoirs about the process of becoming a professional chef; two examples among many are Kathleen Flinn's *The Sharper Your Knife, The Less You Cry* (2007) and Katherine Darling's *Under the Table* (2009). Some readers may not be aware, though, of the memoirs others have written about what it is actually like to work night-by-night in a restaurant; Debra Ginsberg's *Waiting* (2001) and Phoebe Damrosch's *Service Included* (2008) are splendid representations.

One of the most interesting memoirs in the restaurant worker subgenre is Pete Jordan's *Dishwasher* (2007), which pays close attention to an often-ignored part of what goes on, usually unseen, at any establishment that serves food. Jordan attempted to get a job washing dishes in all fifty states, and (prior to the era of social media) had been publishing a *Dishwasher* 'zine that received fan mail from other restaurant dishwashers, some of which is included in the back pages of his book. On the one hand, as Jordan himself acknowledges, his narrative can't pretend to speak for the thousands of underpaid, sometimes non-English speaking immigrants who may end up doing the same job, although as the youngest of five kids with an immigrant father who never finished high school, he is aware of what it means not to have money or privilege. During most of his days as a dishwasher, he only manages to eat by scrounging whatever he can from the unfinished plates of food that come into the dishroom. On the other hand, Jordan's memoir is fascinating for the purposes of "reading one's plate" because his narrative is concerned with exactly that. Throughout the book, he tells us what he scrapes off of the plates (and sometimes eats) during his job, such as garlic bread and crème brulée. This is another way of asking the reader to pay close attention not just to what one eats, but to all of the issues of labor, waste, social class, and hunger that are there behind the scenes. And again, his act of transforming his experience into prose is an instructive example of the intersections between the materialities of cuisine and of literary narrative.

I close the third portion of this after-dinner chapter by offering what every meal should end with: namely, ice cream. To do this, I will turn briefly to a short piece by Sarah DiGregorio, originally published on Gilt-Taste.com and republished in *Best Food Writing 2013*, entitled "When There Was Nothing Left to Do, I Fed Her Ice Cream." DiGregorio begins with her mother's "uncomplicated relationship with ice cream": she ate it, without guilt, whenever she could, sometimes even as a meal in itself (DiGregorio 2013, 371). In later years, when her mother was dying of cancer and was no longer able to experience other pleasures such as reading, her love for ice cream remained, and DiGregorio fed her cup after cup of it: "I couldn't stop dishing out those Hoodsie cups, like they were some kind of sweet miracle drug, and she never stopped me" (DiGregorio 2013, 372). The author wonders whether the ice cream caused her mother on some subconscious level to recall cranking a wooden ice cream machine in the summertime as a child, but says she never asked. Rereading DiGregorio's essay resonated profoundly for me on a personal level because my own mother, who suffered from vascular dementia and lost many of her cognitive skills in the months before her death, never ceased to take profound pleasure in eating those little cups of ice cream that they served in the nursing home—and like DiGregorio, in an odd reversal of mother/daughter roles, she preferred having me feed them to her even though she was more or less capable of eating them by herself. Considering this image, for me, thus brings together so many of the ingredients I have mentioned in the course of this study: the connections between food and memory, the presence of the iconic and significant food object, the complicated parent-child relationship, and—finally—the persistence of hunger, not just for food but for the interpretation of narrative.

Bibliography

Abu-Jaber, Diana. 2005. *The Language of Baklava*. New York: Anchor.
———. 2016. *Life without a Recipe*. New York: W.W. Norton.
Adams, Carol J. 1990. *The Sexual Politics of Meat*. New York: Continuum.
———. 2018. *Burger*. New York and London: Bloomsbury.
Antin, Eleanor. 1981. "Carving: A Traditional Sculpture." *High Performance* 4 (Winter 1981–1982).
Arsenault, Rachel. 2015. "Tourtière: A French-Canadian Meat Pie Recipe." http://www.growagoodlife.com/tourtiere/. December 14, 2015. Accessed July 30, 2018.
Backes, Nancy. 1989. "Body Art: Hunger and Satiation in the Plays of Tina Howe." In *Making a Spectacle: Feminist Essays on Contemporary Women's Theatre*, edited by Lynda Hart, 41–60. Ann Arbor: University of Michigan Press.
Barthes, Roland. 1972. *Mythologies*. Trans. Annette Lavers. New York: Farrar, Straus, Giroux.
Bennett, Jane. 2010. *Vibrant Matter: A Political Ecology of Things*. Durham, NC: Duke University Press. Kindle Edition.
Berger, John. 1972. *Ways of Seeing*. Middlesex, England: Penguin Press/BBC.
Billington, Michael. 2004. "Theatre: Calcutta Kosher: Southwark Playhouse, London" [Review]. *The Guardian*, February 7, 2004.
Birringer, Johannes. 1993. "Imprints and Re-Visions: Carolee Schneeman's Visual Archaeology." *Performing Arts Journal* 15 (May 1993): 31–46.
Blake, William. 1977. *Songs of Innocence and Experience*. 1789–1794. Oxford: Oxford University Press.
Bogost, Ian. 2012. *Alien Phenomenology, Or What It's Like to Be a Thing*. Minneapolis: University of Minnesota Press.
Bollinger, Heidi Elizabeth. 2014. "The Danger of Rereading: Disastrous Endings in Paul Auster's *The Brooklyn Follies* and Jhumpa Lahiri's *Unaccustomed Earth*." *Studies in the Novel* 46, no.4 (Winter 2014): 486–506.
Bordo, Susan. 1993. *Unbearable Weight: Feminism, Western Culture, and the Body*. Berkeley: University of California Press.
Bosmajian, Hamida. 2003. "The Orphaned Voice in Art Spiegelman's *Maus*." In *Considering Maus: Approaches to Art Spiegelman's "Survivor's Tale" of the Holocaust*, edited by Deborah R. Geis, 26–43. Tuscaloosa: University of Alabama Press.
Bourdain, Anthony. 2000. *Kitchen Confidential: Adventures in the Culinary Underbelly*. Revised edition. New York: HarperCollins.
———. 2001. *A Cook's Tour*. New York: Bloomsbury USA.
———. 2006. *The Nasty Bits: Collected Varietal Cuts, Usable Trim, Scraps, and Bones*. New York: Bloomsbury USA.
———. 2007. *No Reservations: Around the World on an Empty Stomach*. New York: Bloomsbury USA.
———. 2010. *Medium Raw: A Bloody Valentine to the World of Food and the People Who Cook*. New York: HarperCollins.
Bourdieu, Pierre. 1984. *Distinction: A Social Critique of the Judgement of Taste*. Trans. Richard Nice. Cambridge, MA: Harvard University Press.
Bower, Anne L. 2009. "Recipes for History: The National Council of Negro Women's Five Historical Cookbooks." In *African American Foodways: Explorations of History & Culture*, edited by Anne L. Bower, 153–74. Urbana & Chicago: University of Illinois Press.

Brown, Bill, ed. 2004. *Things*. Chicago: University of Chicago Press.

Bruni, Frank. 2009. *Born Round*. New York: Penguin Press.

Butler, Judith. 1990. *Gender Trouble*. New York and London: Routledge.

Campbell-Schmitt, Adam. 2018. "Chefs React to Anthony Bourdain's Death." http://www.foodandwine.com/news/anthony-bourdain-death-chef-reactions. June 8, 2018. Accessed July 23, 2018.

Capon, Robert Farrar. 2015. "from *The Supper of the Lamb*: On the Onion." In *Eating Words*, edited by Sandra M. Gilbert and Roger J. Porter, 204–10. New York: W.W. Norton.

Case, Sue Ellen. 1988. *Feminism and Theatre*. New York and London: Methuen.

Chapman, Sasha. 2018. "Tourtière." http://www.britannica.com/topic/tourtiere. July 18, 2018. Accessed July 30, 2018.

Chernin, Kim. 1981. *The Obsession: Reflections on the Tyranny of Slenderness*. New York: Harper/Perennial.

———. 1985. *The Hungry Self: Women, Eating, and Identity*. New York: Harper/Perennial.

Chicago, Judy. 1977. *Through the Flower: My Struggle as a Woman Artist*. New York: Doubleday.

Chin, Ava. 2014. *Eating Wildly: Foraging for Life, Love, and the Perfect Meal*. New York: Simon & Schuster.

Chodorow, Nancy. 1978. *The Reproduction of Mothering: Psychoanalysis and the Sociology of Gender*. Berkeley: University of California Press.

Chopin, Kate. 2017. *The Awakening*. New York: W.W. Norton.

Coetzee, J.M. 2000. "Messages and Silence" [book review]. *New York Review of Books*, May 25, 2000.

Cooke, Nathalie. 2009. *What's to Eat? Entrées in Canadian Food History*. Montréal: McGill-Queen's University Press.

Cooper, Zaki. 2006. "Tolerance, Integration, and Kosher Curry." *The Times* (London), August 26, 2006.

Coward, Rosalind. 1985. *Female Desires: How They Are Sought, Bought, and Packaged*. New York: Grove Press.

Curtin, Deane W. 1992. "Food/Body/Person." In *Cooking, Eating, Thinking: Transformative Philosophies of Food*, edited by Deane W. Curtin and Lisa M. Heldke, 3–22. Bloomington: Indiana University Press.

Curtis, Nick. 2004. "Family in a Pickle" [Review]. *The Evening Standard*, June 15, 2004.

Damrosch, Phoebe. 2008. *Service Included: Four-Star Secrets of an Eavesdropping Waiter*. New York: Harper.

Darling, Katherine. 2009. *Under the Table: Saucy Tales from Culinary School*. New York: Atria.

de Silva, Cara, ed. 1996. *In Memory's Kitchen: A Legacy from the Women of Terezín*. Lanham, MD: Rowman & Littlefield.

Desai, Anita. 1988. *Baumgartner's Bombay*. Boston: Houghton Mifflin.

———. 2000. *Fasting, Feasting*. Boston: Houghton Mifflin.

DiGregorio, Sarah. 2013. "When There Was Nothing Left to Do, I Fed Her Ice Cream." In *Best Food Writing 2013*, edited by Holly Hughes, 371–73. Boston: DaCapo Press.

Douglass, Frederick. 1995. *Narrative of the Life of Frederick Douglass*. New York: Dover Publications.

Eagleton, Terry. 2015. "Edible Ecriture." In *Eating Words*, edited by Sandra M. Gilbert and Roger J. Porter, 445–49. New York: W.W. Norton.

Elias, Megan J. 2017. *Food on the Page: Cookbooks and American Culture*. Philadelphia: University of Pennsylvania Press.

Esquivel, Laura. 1995. *Like Water for Chocolate: A Novel in Monthly Installments with Recipes, Romances, and Home Remedies*. Trans. Carol Christensen and Thomas Christensen. New York: Anchor.

"*Fasting, Feasting*" [book review]. 1999. *Publishers Weekly*, December 6, 1999.

Ferguson, Priscilla Parkhurst. 2014. *Word of Mouth: What We Talk About When We Talk About Food*. Berkeley: University of California Press.

Fernández-Arnesto, Felipe. 2015. "from *Near a Thousand Tables*: The Logic of Cannibalism." In *Eating Words*, edited by Sandra M. Gilbert and Roger J. Porter, 336–45. New York: W.W. Norton.

Fine, Gary A. 1996. *Kitchens: The Culture of Restaurant Work*. Berkeley: University of California Press.

Fine, Laura. 2011. "Space and Hybridity in Jhumpa Lahiri's 'Unaccustomed Earth' and 'Only Goodness.'" *South Asian Review* 32, no. 2: 209–22.

Finley, Karen. 1988. *The Constant State of Desire. TDR* 32 (Spring 1988).

———. 1990. *Shock Treatment*. San Francisco: City Lights Books, 1990.

Fisher, M.F.K. 1942. *How to Cook a Wolf*. New York: North Point Press.

———. 1943. *The Gastronomical Me*. New York: North Point Press.

———. 1949. *An Alphabet for Gourmets*. New York: North Point Press.

———. 1990. *The Art of Eating*. New York: Collier Macmillan.

Flinn, Kathleen. 2007. *The Sharper Your Knife, The Less You Cry*. New York: Penguin Press.

Florsheim, Stewart. 1989. "Weekend in Palm Springs." In *Ghosts of the Holocaust: An Anthology of Poetry by the Second Generation*, 78–79. Detroit: Wayne State University Press.

Foer, Jonathan Safran. 2009. *Eating Animals*. New York: Little, Brown.

Forte, Jeanie. 1992. "Focus on the Body: Pain, Praxis, and Pleasure in Feminist Performance." *Critical Theory and Performance*, edited by Janelle G. Reinelt and Joseph R. Roach. Ann Arbor: University of Michigan Press.

Furiya, Linda. 2006. *Bento Box in the Heartland: My Japanese Girlhood in Whitebread America*. Berkeley, CA: Seal Press.

———. 2008. *How to Cook a Dragon: Living, Loving, and Eating in China*. Berkeley, CA: Seal Press.

Fuss, Diana. 1998. "A Supper Party." In *Eating Culture*, edited by Ron Scapp and Brian Seitz, 237–43. Albany: SUNY Press.

Fussell, Betty. 2015. "Eating My Words." In *Eating Words*, edited by Sandra M. Gilbert and Roger J. Porter, 439–44. New York: W.W. Norton.

Gajanan, Mahita. 2018. "Anthony Bourdain Remembered as an 'Unabashedly Supportive' Advocate and Ally in #MeToo." http://www.foodandwine.com/syndication/anthony-bourdain-metoo. June 8, 2018. Accessed July 23, 2018.

Garner, Stanton B., Jr. 1994. *Bodied Spaces: Phenomenology and Performance in Contemporary Drama*. Ithaca: Cornell University Press.

Gates Jr., Henry Louis. 2015. "from *Colored People*: Wet Dogs and White People." In *Eating Words*, edited by Sandra M. Gilbert and Roger J. Porter, 156–60. New York: W.W. Norton.

Geis, Deborah R. 1993. *Postmodern Theatric(k)s: Monologue in Contemporary American Drama*. Ann Arbor: University of Michigan Press.

———. 2008. *Suzan-Lori Parks*. Ann Arbor: University of Michigan Press.

Gilbert, Elizabeth. 2007. *Eat, Pray, Love*. New York: Riverhead.

Gilbert, Sandra M. 2014. *The Culinary Imagination: From Myth to Modernity*. New York: W.W. Norton.

Gilbert, Sandra M. and Roger J. Porter. 2015. "Introduction: A Toast to Taste." In *Eating Words*, edited by Sandra M. Gilbert and Roger J. Porter, xxv–xxxiii. New York: W.W. Norton.

Ginsberg, Allen. 2006. *Collected Poems 1947–1997*. New York: Harper Perennial.

Ginsberg, Debra. 2001. *Waiting: The True Confessions of a Waitress*. New York: Harper Perennial.

Gopnik, Adam. 2015. "from What's the Recipe? Our Hunger for Cookbooks." In *Eating Words*, edited by Sandra M. Gilbert and Roger J. Porter, 456–64. New York: W.W. Norton.

Gordon, Mel. 1983. *Lazzi: The Comic Routines of the Commedia dell'Arte*. New York: Performing Arts Journal Publications.

Halliday, Ayun. 2006. *Dirty Sugar Cookies*. Emeryville, CA: Seal Press.

Hamalian, Linda. 1986. "Allen Ginsberg in the Eighties" [interview]. *Literary Review* 29, no. 3 (March 1986): 293–300.

Hamilton, Gabrielle. 2011. *Blood, Bones & Butter: The Inadvertent Education of a Reluctant Chef*. New York: Random House.

Harris, Jessica B. 1996. *The Welcome Table: African American Heritage Cooking*. New York: Simon & Schuster.

———. 2012. *High on the Hog: A Culinary Journey from Africa to America*. New York: Bloomsbury USA.

Hass, Aaron. 1990. *In the Shadow of the Holocaust*. Ithaca: Cornell University Press; rpt. Cambridge: Cambridge University Press, 1996.

———. 1996. *The Aftermath: Living with the Holocaust*. Cambridge: Cambridge University Press.

Hayes, Terrance. 2002. "Sonnet." *Hip Logic*, 13. New York: Penguin Press.

Henderson, Jeff and Ramin Ganeshram, eds. 2011. *America I AM: Pass it Down Cookbook*. New York: Smiley/Bayhouse.

Henderson, Jeff. 2007. *Cooked: My Journey from the Streets to the Stove*. New York: Harper.

Henri, Adrian. 1974. *Total Art: Environments, Happenings, and Performance*. Oxford and New York: Oxford University Press.

hooks, bell. 1998. "Eating the Other: Desire and Resistance." In *Eating Culture*, edited by Ron Scapp and Brian Seitz, 181–200. Albany: SUNY Press.

Husserl, Edmund. 2013. *Ideas: General Introduction to Pure Phenomenology*. 1931. Trans. W. R. Boyce Gibson. New York: Routledge.

Hyman, Mavis. 1992. *Indian-Jewish Cooking*. London: Longdunn.

Jameson, Fredric. 1991. *Postmodernism, or The Cultural Logic of Late Capitalism*. Durham: Duke University Press.

Johnson, Barbara. 2003. *Mother Tongues: Sexuality, Trials, Motherhood, Translation*. Cambridge, MA: Harvard University Press.

Jordan, Pete. 2007. *Dishwasher*. New York: Harper Perennial.

Jordan, Rayna. 2018. "French Canadian Tourtière." http://www.allrecipes.com/recipe/20752/french-canadian-tourtiere . Accessed July 30, 2018.

Juno, Andrea. 1991. Interview with Karen Finley. In *Re/Search #13: Angry Women*, edited by Andrea Juno and V. Vale. San Francisco: Re/Search Publications.

Kerouac, Jack. 1991. *The Dharma Bums*. New York: Penguin Press.

Kinsman, Kat. 2018. "We Need to Talk about Anthony Bourdain." http://www.foodandwine.com/chefs/anthony-bourdain. June 8, 2018. Accessed July 23, 2018.

Kristeva, Julia. 1980. *Desire in Language*. Trans. by Thomas Gora, Alice Jardine, and Leon S. Roudiez. New York: Columbia University Press.

Lahiri, Jhumpa. 2000. "Indian Takeout." Originally appeared in *Food and Wine Magazine*. In *Eating Words: A Norton Anthology of Food Writing*, edited by Sandra M. Gilbert and Roger J. Porter, 183–86. New York: W.W. Norton.

———. 2004. "The Long Way Home." *New Yorker*, September 6, 2004.

———. 2009. *Unaccustomed Earth*. New York: Vintage Books.

Lakshmi, Padma. 2016. *Love, Loss, and What We Ate*. New York: Ecco Press.

Levine, Michael G. 2003. "Necessary Stains: Art Spiegelman's *Maus* and the Bleeding of History." In *Considering Maus: Approaches to Art Spiegelman's "Survivor's Tale" of the Holocaust*, edited by Deborah R. Geis, 63–104. Tuscaloosa: University of Alabama Press.

Lippard, Lucy. 1988. "Lacy: Some of Her Own Medicine." *TDR* 32 (Spring 1988): 71–76.

Louis, Yvette. 2001. "Body Language: The Black Female Body and the Word in Suzan-Lori Parks's *The Death of the Last Black Man in the Whole Entire World*." In *Recovering the Black Female Body: Self-Representations by African American Women*, edited by Michael Bennett and Vanessa D. Dickerson, 141–64. New Brunswick: Rutgers University Press.

Lugones, María. 1992. "Playfulness, 'World'-Travelling, and Loving Perception." In *Cooking, Eating, Thinking: Transformative Philosophies of Food*, edited by Deane W. Curtin and Lisa M. Heldke, 85–99. Bloomington: Indiana University Press.

MacClancy, Jeremy. 1992. *Consuming Culture*. London: Chapman.

Manring, M.M. 1998. *Slave in a Box: The Strange Career of Aunt Jemima*. Charlottesville: University of Virginia Press.

Margulies, Donald. 1995. *"The Model Apartment."* In *Sight Unseen and Other Plays*, 142–95. New York: Theatre Communications Group.

Marinetti, F.T. 1989. *The Futurist Cookbook*, edited by Lesley Chamberlain. Trans. Suzanne Brill. San Francisco: Bedford Arts.

Miller, Nancy K. 2003. "Cartoons of the Self: Portrait of the Artist as a Young Murderer—Art Spiegelman's *Maus*." In *Considering MAUS: Approaches to Art Spiegelman's "Survivor's Tale" of the Holocaust*, edited by Deborah R. Geis, 44–59. Tuscaloosa: University of Alabama Press.

Milton, John. 2010. *Paradise Lost*. New York: Signet Books.

Mitchell, Elvis. 2010. "A Conversation with Anthony Bourdain." In *Medium Raw: A Bloody Valentine to the World of Food and the People Who Cook*, by Anthony Bourdain, Backmatter ("P.S."). New York: HarperCollins.

Montano, Linda. 1981. "Food and Art" [interviews]. *High Performance* 4 (Winter 1981–1982).

Morgan, Bill. 2007. *I Celebrate Myself: The Somewhat Private Life of Allen Ginsberg*. New York: Penguin Press.

Morton, Timothy. 2013. *Realist Magic: Objects, Ontology, Causality*. Ann Arbor: MPublishing.

Moses, Kate. 2010. *Cakewalk: A Memoir*. New York: Dial Press.

Mulvey, Laura. 1995. "Visual Pleasure and Narrative Cinema." Orig. 1975. In *Feminist Film Theory: A Reader*, edited by Sue Thornham, 58–69. New York: New York University Press.

Nadotti, Maria. 1989. "Karen Finley's Poisoned Meatloaf." Trans. Meg Shore. *Artforum* 27 (March 1989): 113.

Narayan, Shoba. 2004. *Monsoon Diary: A Memoir with Recipes*. New York: Random House.

Neary, Lynn. 2011. "Tourtière: A French-Canadian Twist on Christmas Pie." "The Salt." http://www.npr.org./sections/thesalt/2014. December 23, 2011. Accessed July 31, 2018.

Nguyen, Bich Minh. 2007. *Stealing Buddha's Dinner*. New York: Viking.

Nightingale, Benedict. 2004. "Cinders without the Sparkle" [Review]. *The Times* (London), February 10, 2004.

Notaker, Henry. 2017. *A History of Cookbooks: From Kitchen to Page Over Seven Centuries*. Berkeley: University of California Press.

O'Neill, Molly. 2015. "from Food Porn." In *Eating Words*, edited by Sandra M. Gilbert and Roger J. Porter, 449–56. New York: W.W. Norton.

Oliver, Kelly. 1992. "Nourishing the Speaking Subject: A Psychoanalytic Approach to Abominable Food and Women." In *Cooking, Eating, Thinking: Transformative Philosophies of Food*, edited by Deane W. Curtin and Lisa M. Heldke, 68–84. Bloomington: Indiana University Press.

Orbach, Susie. 1978. *Fat is a Feminist Issue*. New York: Berkley/Paddington.

Parker, Mike. 2004. "Touching, Comic Clash of Cultures" [Review]. *Morning Star*, July 1, 2004.

Parks, Suzan-Lori. 1995a. *"The Death of the Last Black Man in the Whole Entire World."* In *The America Play and Other Works*, 100–31. New York: Theatre Communications Group.

——. 1995b. "*Pickling*." In *The America Play and Other Works*, 93–98. New York: Theatre Communications Group.

——. 1997. *Venus*. New York: Theatre Communications Group.

——. 2001a. *The Red Letter Plays* [*In the Blood* and *Fucking A*]. New York: Theatre Communications Group.

——. 2001b. *Topdog/Underdog*. New York: Theatre Communications Group.

——. 2015. *Father Comes Home from the Wars, Parts 1, 2, & 3*. New York: Theatre Communications Group.

Patraka, Vivian. 1992. "Binary Terror and Feminist Performance: Reading Both Ways." *Discourse* 14 (Spring 1992): 163–85.

——. 1999. *Spectacular Suffering: Theatre, Fascism, and the Holocaust*. Bloomington: Indiana University Press.

Persley, Nicole Hodges. 2010. "Sampling and Remixing: Hip Hop and Parks's History Plays." In *Suzan-Lori Parks: Essays on the Plays and Other Works*, edited by Philip C. Kolin, 65–75. Jefferson, NC: McFarland.

Peter, John. 2004. "Rest of the Week's Theatre: Calcutta Kosher" [Review]. *The Sunday Times* (London), February 15, 2004.

Peyton, Gabby. 2018. "Iconic Canadian Food: Tourtière—Canada's Meat Pie." http://www.foodbloggersofcanada.com/tourtiere-canadas-meat-pie. Accessed July 31, 2018.

Pollan, Michael. 2006. *The Omnivore's Dilemma*. New York: Penguin Press.

——. 2008. *In Defense of Food: An Eater's Manifesto*. New York: Penguin Press.

Poon, Angelia. 2008. "In a Transnational World: Exploring Gendered Subjectivity, Mobility, and Consumption in Anita Desai's *Fasting, Feasting*." *Ariel* 37, nos. 2–3 (April 2008): 33–48.

Popkin, Barry. 2009. *The World Is Fat: The Fads, Trends, Policies and Products That Are Fattening the Human Race*. New York: Avery/Penguin Group.

Powell, Julie. 2005. *Julie and Julia*. New York: Little, Brown.

——. 2009. *Cleaving: A Story of Marriage, Meat, and Obsession*. New York: Little, Brown.

Prose, Francine. 2000. "Let Them Eat Curry" [book review]. *New York Times Book Review*, January 9, 2000.

Reichl, Ruth. 1998. *Tender at the Bone*. New York: Broadway.

——. 2001. *Comfort Me with Apples*. New York: Random House.

——. 2005. *Garlic and Sapphires: The Secret Life of a Critic in Disguise*. New York: Penguin Press.

——. 2010. *For You, Mom, Finally*. New York: Penguin Press.

"Remarks on Parks 2." 2006. Hunter College Symposium on Suzan-Lori Parks: Directors. http://www.hotreview.org/articles/Remarksparks2.htm. Accessed January 19, 2006.

Reynolds, Jonathan. *Wrestling with Gravy*. 2006. New York: Random House.

Ritzer, George, ed. 2002. *McDonaldization: The Reader*. Thousand Oaks, CA: Pine Forge Press.

Rosner, Elizabeth. 1998. "Disobedient Child." *Gravity*, 35. Concord, CA: Small Poetry Press.

Roth, Moira. 1988. "Suzanne Lacy: Social Reformer and Witch." *TDR* 32 (Spring 1988): 42–60.

Samuelsson, Marcus. 2012. *Yes, Chef: A Memoir*. New York: Random House.

Sayre, Henry M. 1989. *The Object of Performance: The American Avant-Garde Since 1970*. Chicago: University of Chicago Press.

Schenone, Laura. 2008. *The Lost Ravioli Recipes of Hoboken*. New York: W.W. Norton.

Schlosser, Eric. 2012. *Fast Food Nation: The Dark Side of the All-American Meal*. Revised ed. New York: Mariner Books.

Shakespeare, William. 2017. *Titus Andronicus*. New York: Penguin Press.

Shange, Ntozake. 1997. *for colored girls who have considered suicide/when the rainbow is enuf*. New York: Charles Scribner.

———. 1998. *if I can Cook/you KNow God can*. Boston: Beacon Press.

———. 2010. *Sassafrass, Cypress & Indigo*. New York: St. Martin's Press.

Shapiro, Laura. 2009. *Perfection Salad: Women and Cooking at the Turn of the Century*. Berkeley: University of California Press.

Silas, Shelby. 2004. *Calcutta Kosher*. London: Oberon.

Skloot, Robert. 1988. *The Darkness We Carry: The Drama of the Holocaust*. Madison: University of Wisconsin Press.

Smart-Grosvenor, Vertamae. 1992. "from *Vibration Cooking: or The Travel Notes of a Geechee Girl*." In *Cooking, Eating, Thinking: Transformative Philosophies of Food*, edited by Deane W. Curtin and Lisa M. Heldke, 294–97. Bloomington: Indiana University Press.

Smith, Dinitia. 1997. "For the Holocaust 'Second Generation,' an Artistic Quest." *New York Times*, December 23, 1997.

Sobell, Nina. 1981. *Baby Chicky* (in "Artists' Portfolio"). *High Performance* 4 (Winter 1981–1982).

Spiegelman, Art. 1986. *Maus I: A Survivor's Tale*. New York: Pantheon.

———. 1991. *Maus II: And Here My Troubles Began*. New York: Pantheon.

Spitz, Bob. 2008. *The Saucier's Apprentice: One Long Strange Trip Through the Great Cooking Schools of Europe*. New York: W.W. Norton.

Steinberg, Stephen. 1998. "Bubbie's Challah." In *Eating Culture*, edited by Ron Scapp and Brian Seitz, 295–97. Albany: SUNY Press.

Sunée, Kim. 2008. *Trail of Crumbs: Hunger, Love, and the Search for Home*. New York: Grand Central.

Thorne, John. 2015. "from *The Outlaw Cook*: Cuisine Mécanique." In *Eating Words*, edited by Sandra M. Gilbert and Roger J. Porter, 278–85. New York: W.W. Norton.

Tisdale, Sallie. 2000. *The Best Thing I Ever Tasted: The Secret of Food*. New York: Riverhead.

Twitty, Michael W. 2017. *The Cooking Gene: A Journey Through African American Culinary History in the Old South*. New York: Amistad/Harper Collins.

Volná, Ludmila. 2005. "Anita Desai's *Fasting, Feasting* and the Condition of Women." *Comparative Literature and Culture* 7, no. 3 (September 2005): 42–50.

Whalen-Bridge, John. 2016. "*Howl* and the Performance of Communion." In *Beat Drama: Playwrights and Performances of the "Howl" Generation*, edited by Deborah R. Geis, 25–31. London and New York: Bloomsbury.

Whit, William C. 2009. "Soul Food as Cultural Creation." In *African American Foodways: Explorations of History and Culture*, edited by Anne L. Bower, 45–58. Urbana: University of Illinois Press.

Whitman, Walt. 2004. *The Complete Poems*. New York and London: Penguin Press.

Williams-Forson, Psyche A. 2006. *Building Houses Out of Chicken Legs: Black Women, Food, & Power*. Chapel Hill: University of North Carolina Press.

Wilson, August. 1992. *Two Trains Running*. New York: E.P. Dutton..

Witt, Doris. 1999. *Black Hunger: Soul Food and America*. Minneapolis: University of Minnesota Press.

Woolf, Virginia. 1989. *To the Lighthouse*. New York: Harcourt Brace.

Wutz, Michael. 2015. "The Archaeology of the Colonial: Unearthing Jhumpa Lahiri's *Unaccustomed Earth*." *Studies in American Fiction* 42, no. 2 (Fall 2015): 243–60.

Yentsch, Anne. 2009. "Excavating the South's African American Food History." In *African American Foodways: Explorations of History and Culture*, edited by Anne L. Bower, 59–98. Urbana: University of Illinois Press.

Zweig, Ellen. 1981. "Fear of Dining and Dining Conversation." *High Performance* 4 (Winter 1981–1982).

Index

About the Author

Deborah R. Geis is professor of English at DePauw University in Greencastle, Indiana, where she specializes in twentieth and twenty-first century literature, particularly drama, performance poetry, African American and Beat Generation literature, and the literature of food. Her previous books include *Postmodern Theatric(k)s*, *Suzan-Lori Parks*, and three edited collections: *Approaching the Millennium: Essays on Angels in America* (co-edited by Steven F. Kruger); *Considering MAUS: Approaches to Art Spiegelman's "Survivor's Tale" of the Holocaust*; and *Beat Drama: Playwrights and Performances of the "Howl" Generation*.